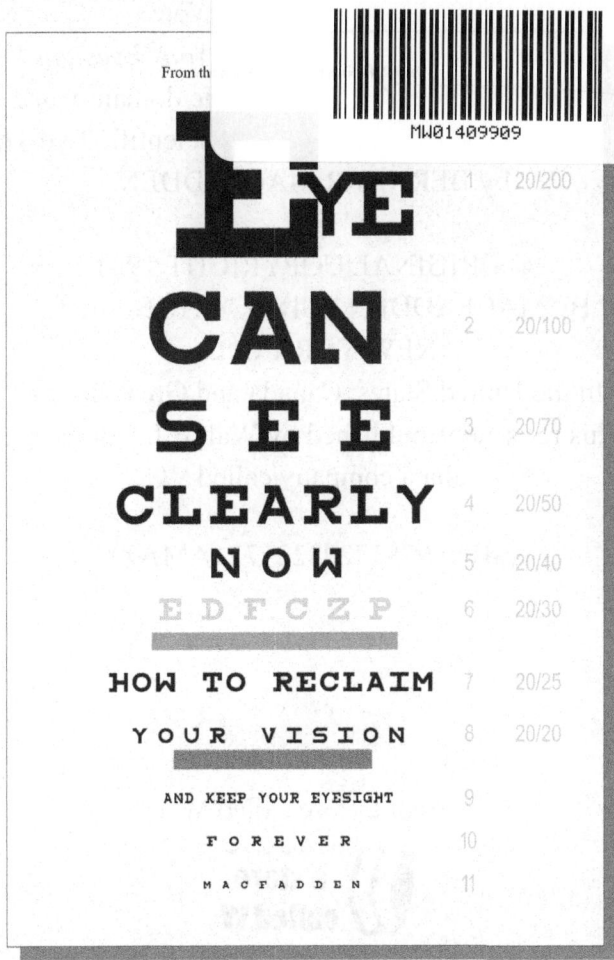

The modern re-issue of the public domain work
Strengthening the EYES
A System of Scientific Eye Training
Bernarr Macfadden

Produced by Walt F.J. Goodridge (aka The Ageless Adept)
the publisher of *Fast & Grow Young*

Eye Can See Clearly Now
How to Reclaim Your Vision and Keep Your Eyesight Forever
The modern re-issue of the public domain work
Strengthening the EYES: A System of Scientific Eye Training
by BERNARR MACFADDEN

><

© ORIGINAL COPYRIGHT 1924
By MACFADDEN PUBLICATIONS, INC.
NEW YORK CITY
In the United States, Canada and Great Britain
This re-issue is published by Walt F.J. Goodridge
dba a company called W

ISBN: 9781720822172 (AMAZ)

Visit a store called W

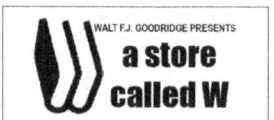

Books, apps, audio, video, merchandise,
courses, Walt's passion projects, freebies
and more from a company called W!
www.waltgoodridge.com/store

Distributed by The Passion Profit Company
Educational institutions, government agencies, libraries and
corporations are invited to inquire about quantity discounts at
(646) 481-4238 | sales@passionprofit.com

Paperback printed in the United States of America

TABLE OF CONTENTS

Publisher's Foreword 6
Original Author's Preface 7
List of Illustrations 10
I. Strong, Beautiful Eyes 13
II. The Anatomy Of The Human Eye 17
III. How We See: Physiology & Physics Of Vision 23
IV. Asthenopia: Weak Eyes 31
V. The Imperfect Sight Of The Normal Eye 33
VI. Errors Of Refraction: Their Cause 37
VII. Errors Of Refraction: Their Cure 41
VIII. Amblyopia 49
IX. Color Blindness 51
X. Strabismus: Squint 53
XI. Saving The Sight Of The Children 55
XII. Common Diseases Of The Eye 61
XIII. Injuries To The Eye 71
XIV. Eye Exercises 73
XV. Eye-Focusing Exercises 78
XVI. Exercises For The Pupil Of The Eye 82
XVII. Eye Massage And Resistance 84
XVIII. The Eye Bath 88
XIX. Eye Strength Through Sunlight 92
XX. Constitutional Improvement For Strengthening The Eyes 95
XXI. Exercises For Constitutional Improvement 98
XXII. Eating For Health And Strength 110
XXIII. Eye Rest Through Sleep 115
XXIV. Fresh Air, Bathing And Other Health Factors 118
XXV. Eye Hygiene 122
XXVI. Test Your Own Eyes 125
XXVII. A Final Word To Those Who Wear Glasses 129
About the Original Author 131
Appendix & Resources 132-140

LIST OF ILLUSTRATIONS

Chap-Fig No. Description Page No.
2-1 Sectional View of the Eye 17
2-2 Diagram of Retina 18
2-3 Muscles and Arteries of Eye 19
2-4 Section Through Right Eye 20
3-1 Illustrating Refraction of Light 24
3-2 Refraction of Light-rays Becoming Divergent 24
3-3 Refraction of Light-rays Becoming Convergent 25
3-4 Refraction of Light-rays from Distant and Nearby Points 26
3-5 Diagram for Demonstrating Blind Spot 27
3-6 Diagram Illustrating Far-sightedness 27
3-7 Diagram Illustrating Near-sightedness 28
3-8 The Lens Not a Factor in Change of Focus (Carp experiment) 28
3-9 Astigmatism Following Change in Shape of Eyeball 29
7-1 Diagram Illustrating Central Fixation 42
7-2 Palming to Relax Eye Strain 44
7-3 Normal Vision and Forced Astigmatism 47
7-4 Seeing Without Strain 48
10-1 Typical Case of Squint or "Cross Eyes" 54
10-2 Squint or "Cross Eyes" Cured 54
11-1 Case of divergent vertical squint 56
11-2 Cure of vertical squint 58
11-3 One Part of Treatment for Squint 58
13-1 Method of Removing Cinders, etc. 72
14-1 Exercising Eye Muscles: Looking left 73
14-2 Exercising Eye Muscles: Looking Right 74
14-3 Exercising Eye Muscles; Looking Upward 74
14-4 Exercising Eye Muscles; Looking Downward 74
14-5 Exercising Eye Muscles; Looking Upward, Obliquely to Left 74
14-6 Exercising Eye Muscles; Looking Downward, Obliquely to Right 74
14-7 Exercising Eye Muscles; Looking Upward, Obliquely to Right 75
14-8 Exercising Eye Muscles; Stretching Obliquely, Downward to Left 75
14-9 Exercising Eye Muscles; Rolling the Eyes 75
14-10 Exercising Eye Muscles; Squeezing Closed Eyelids 75
14-11 Exercising Eye Muscles; Looking Cross-eyed 75
14-12 Diagram for Exercising the Eyes 79
14-13 A Second Diagram for Exercising the Eyes 79
14-14 A Third Diagram for Exercising the Eyes 79
15-1 Eye-focusing Exercise for Both Eyes 81
15-2 Eye-focusing Exercise; Using Eyes Alternatively 81
15-3 Eye-focusing Exercise; Closing and Opening the Eye 82
15-4 Combination Eyeball and Eye-focusing Exercise 82
15-5 Another Form of Eyeball and Eye-focusing Exercise 82

16-1 Exercising the Pupil of the Eye 84
17-1 Using Heel of Hand for Eye Massage 85
17-2 Using Thum and Finger for Eye Massage 85
17-3 Another Form of Eye Massage 85
17-4 A Gentle Resistance Exercise for Eyes 86
17-5 Another Form of Resistance Exercise for Eyes 86
18-1 Wash Bowl for Taking Eye Bath 89
18-2 Taking the Eye Bath in a Basin 89
18-3 The Eye-cup 90
18-4 Taking the Eye Bath With an Eye-Cup 90
19-1 No Injury to Eyes When Looking at the Sun 95
19-2 Reading in Direct Sunlight 96
19-3 Sunlight as an Eye Curative Agent 96
21-1 Exercise for Body; Hips Bent Forward 99
21-2 Exercise for Body; Bending Backward 99
21-3 Exercise for Body; Bending Sideways 99
21-4 Exercise for Body; Twisting from Side to Side 100
21-5 Exercise for Body; Stretch upward 100
21-6 Exercise for Body; Raising Up on Toes 100
21-7 Exercise for Body; Squatting Position 101
21-8 Exercise for Body; Raising Knees 101
21-9 Exercise for Body; Lying on Back Raising Torso 101
21-10 Exercise for Body; Lying on Back, Raising Legs 102
21-11 Exercise for Body; Raising Hips and Back from Floor 102
21-12 Exercise for Body; Lying Face Downward, Raising Feet and Legs 102
21-13 Exercise for Body; Face Downward, Raising Head and Shoulders 102
21-14 Exercise for Body; Squatting and Jumping 103
21-15 Exercise for Body; Raising Body from Toes and Hands 103
21-16 Exercise for Body; Return to crouching position 103
21-17 Exercise for Body; Shadow Boxing 107
21-18 Exercise for Body; A Stationary Run 107
21-19 Exercise for Body; Neck Resistance Exercise 107
21-20 Exercise for Body; Neck Exercise 107
21-21 Exercise for Body; A Simple Neck Exercise 107
21-22,23,24 Exercise for Body; Free Movement Neck Exercise 108
26-1 Testing the Eye With the Retinoscope 125
26-2 A Simple Home-made Retinoscope 127
Snellen Eye Chart 133
Portrait of Author

PUBLISHER'S FOREWORD

*"Truth doesn't expire.
Often it simply falls out of favor."*

Eye Can See Clearly Now is the modern reissue of Bernarr Macfadden's 1924—now public domain--work, Strengthening the EYES A System of Scientific Eye Training, under a new title, with the goal of maintaining public access to this vital information in new formats.

It is a sad fact of our modern existence that practically everything we've been told, taught and led to believe--particularly about the body, health, sickness, and healing--is, quite frankly, wrong. *Don't look at the sun. Glasses can correct your vision. Astigmatism is incurable. Myopia is hereditary*. These and other myths, untruths and even "food crimes" are revealed within the pages of *Eye Can See Clearly Now*. Don't let the original copyright date fool you, truth is timeless. The human body hasn't changed since 1924.

Macfadden's work underscores the Ageless Adept philosophy that the universe is perfect, nature is foolproof, the body is coded to heal and that our access to real and lasting cure exist by design as an instinctive part of natural law as well as that pre-wired, inborn coding. In order to sustain vitality, one need only replicate the earth's original, pristine conditions of sunlight, air, water, sun earth and (real) food.

As insightful as his conclusions are, Macfadden, like many authors, was limited by the worldview of his culture and times. Consequently, certain content may not "pass" today's standards of political correctness. The reader who can make allowances for the biases of his time and dig below a few politically incorrect references, will uncover and rescue the underlying philosophy which is, at its core, unassailable: that in his quest for health and youth, man is best served by natural means. You are your own authority

With that said, I present to you, with minimal editing and spelling corrections to the original text, *Eye Can See Clearly Now!*

--Walt F.J. Goodridge, author of over 24 books including

In Search of a Better Belief System, The Man Who Lived Forever, Fit to Breed...Forever! and *A Clean Cell Never Dies*

ORIGINAL AUTHOR'S PREFACE
▲

Eyes speak all languages; wait for no letter of introduction; they ask no leave of age or rank; they respect neither poverty nor riches; neither learning nor power, nor virtue, nor sex, but intrude and come again, and go through and through you in a moment of time.—Emerson.

Nearly twenty-five years have passed since my interest was aroused in the problem of strengthening the eyes. It was the result of an experience that came near to being tragical.

No one can adequately measure the value of sight; but when we feel it failing we can in some degree realize what that value is. Such was my case on the occasion referred to. At the time I was assuming unusual responsibilities in the editorial and business management of the *PHYSICAL CULTURE MAGAZINE*, the publication having recently leapt into a prominent position, making the work extremely difficult. I had also undertaken to write an important book, the correspondence I was receiving having led me to see that there would be a large demand for the information that I expected to include therein.

Before having done any work on the book, except to divide the important phases of the subject into chapters, I advertised it, thinking it could well be finished and printed, ready for sale, at the time announced. My other duties, however, were so exacting that I was unable to begin writing when I expected to.

The demand for the work was extraordinary; orders poured into the office at the rate of two or three hundred a day, and further delay was out of the question. No one could assume my particular duties in editing and publishing the PHYSICAL CULTURE MAGAZINE; and moreover, at that time I had no assistant editors, or proofreaders, to relieve me of details. Therefore, in order to get any time for the book I was obliged to labor far into the night. By working night and day, however, I was able to finish it in about thirty days.

But the morning after the last corrected proof had been returned to the printer, I was appalled by the condition of my eyes. Vision was imperfect in many ways, and on picking up a newspaper, the printed page appeared like solid black.

I realized in a few seconds the value of my eyesight, and I did some rapid and serious thinking.

I had no faith in oculists and less in other doctors; the thought of consulting them did not even occur to me. I knew that my eyes must have been affected both locally and constitutionally, for not only had they been subjected to extreme overwork, but this overwork had lowered my general vitality. Whatever my business responsibilities might be, I saw that a vacation was now necessary, and I accordingly took it.

After returning to my duties in about two weeks, my eyes were greatly improved, but their condition was still far from satisfactory. I finally concluded to take a fast of one week in order to cleanse thoroughly my physical organism. This benefited my eyes tremendously. Thereafter I began to experiment with various eye exercises together with the eye bath, massage, etc., and my eyes soon acquired their former vigor.

Oculists with whom I came in contact during this period warned me of the dangers of adhering to my views. Blindness, they said, would surely be my fate.

In recent years I have been informed on numerous occasions that the eyes naturally begin to deteriorate after forty years of age, and that total blindness might result if I did not assist them with glasses. About ten years ago (I am now in my fifty-fifth year), when I was treating hundreds of patients at the Bernarr Macfadden Healthatorium in Chicago, one of my patients, an oculist, was very emphatic in his warnings as to the danger I was running by not wearing glasses, and he finally induced me to promise him that I would try a pair if he sent them to me after he returned home. The glasses arrived in due time, but after wearing them for about ten minutes my eyes pained me so severely that I had to discard them. No doubt they were not adjusted to the condition of my eyes, but I did not try to improve upon them. I have refrained from adopting the "eye crutch" up to the present time, and I hope that for many years to come I shall be able to avoid them. As a result of the natural methods of treatment already explained, my eyes are excellent and I work strenuously with both brain and eyes regularly six days per week, and long, tedious days at that

When my book, *Strong Eyes,* was first published, the principles presented therein were to a certain extent new, but I was thoroughly convinced of their correctness and thousands of readers have attested their value since the first edition of the book was issued. More than fifty thousand copies of the book have been sold, and in no instance have I heard of an injury to the eyes because of the use of the methods outlined therein; but, on the other hand, thousands have borne witness to extraordinary benefit derived from them, while numbers have been able to discard their glasses altogether as a result of their use.

Consequently this book is presented, not as a mere set of complex and untried theories, but as an aggregation of definite and practical facts.

Some years ago I came in contact with the work of a prominent eye specialist who is a scientist of high standing in the field of ophthalmology and a graduate of the College of Physicians and Surgeons, Columbia University, New York. This physician began his studies in connection with his revolutionary theories in 1886. It was in this year that he cured his first case of myopia (near-sight). Encouraged by this success, he treated many patients at the New York Eye Infirmary with benefit, accomplishing some complete cures. While he was at the New York Post Graduate, his success was such as to bring about the loss of his position, the eye specialist in charge there maintaining that such cures were impossible, and this notwithstanding the fact that the proof was there for investigation.

In 1903 this physician discovered that teachers could not only prevent the occurrence of myopia among their pupils, but could cure it by the use of the "Snellen test card." This was the first successful method for the prevention of myopia and other cases of imperfect sight in school children, and in itself is a discovery that will greatly benefit humanity. (See New York Medical Journal, July 29, 1911.) In 1912 this method was introduced into some of the public schools of the city of New York, the results being published in the New York Medical Journal, August 30, 1913. The teachers cured one thousand children of imperfect sight without the help of glasses.

During the last ten years, this scientist has made many experiments on rabbits, fish, cats and dogs for the purpose of gaining information about the action of the external muscles of the eye. By this means he has been able to bring to light many facts which are entirely opposite to the theories about the eye published in text books at the present time. These experiments, some details of which may be found in the New York Medical Journal for May 8, 1915, together with his untiring studies of the human eye, have further led this physician to formulate a system of eye training by means of which not only errors of refraction but almost every irregularity of the eye can either be cured or materially benefited without the help of glasses.

Directly opposed to the methods and theories of orthodoxy, this system is not only revolutionary in character, but far-reaching in its practical importance.

I feel sure that in adopting the ideas of this eminent scientist I have been able not only to stamp my own theories with the approval of up-to-date science, but to present to the public a course of eye training which will bear the most searching criticism.

It is scientific and practical, and has been proven conclusively to be of inestimable value. It should enable you to so strengthen your eyes that glasses will not be needed later in life, while in many cases it will enable you to discard the glasses which you may now be wearing; it should also enable many to avoid the loss of a possession priceless in value—the sense of sight.

This book is sent out in the hope that it will be a boon to many who need the invaluable information which it contains. That its methods sometimes require considerable time and patience for their successful practice should not lessen their value. The rewards which await those who follow the instructions given will be beyond price.

"Perfect health, long life and eternal youth are not the random, genetic blessings of a chaotic or capricious universe, but natural birthrights that can be accessed through the mindful acceptance of simple truths, activated by the disciplined practice of proven activities, and sustained by advancement along a known path. This is that path."--**The Ageless Adept**

CHAPTER I:
Strong, Beautiful Eyes ▲

Strong, Beautiful Eyes
Eyes,
Of microscopic power, that would discern
the population of a dewdrop.
—Montgomery.

It is undoubtedly true that man comes into more intimate contact with the outer world through the sense of sight than through any other, or perhaps through all the others combined. In the case of the other senses, outside impressions: or "stimuli" seem to come *to* the man—to impinge *upon* him, as it were; but in the case of sight, he apparently goes outside himself, and actually seems to project himself into the outer world—seeing what is there, actually existing. We know now that this subjective impression of the facts is not true; but the feeling is there none the less. We can also direct or govern the sense of sight more fully than any other. We can "turn away" from sights we do not wish to see, while we cannot readily stop listening to sounds we do not like or shut out smells which are disagreeable to us. Sight seems to be, more than any other sense, in touch with the true personality—the godlike self within.

Yet, in spite of their great value, the eyes are among the most delicate organs in the human body. They are composed largely of liquid, are extremely sensitive, and can very readily be destroyed altogether. It is only the marvelous protective measures of nature which prevent a greater number of fatal injuries to these organs.

Man, more than any other animal, depends upon his sense of sight, for in his case the other senses, such as smell and hearing, are more or less "atrophied," or stunted, as compared with their keenness in other animals. They are sometimes almost lost through lack of use. To a certain extent this is true of the sense of sight also, but it is less true here than in the other instances, the conditions of modern life requiring the almost constant use of the organs of vision.

The eye in the lower animal, as well as in man, is one of the most highly specialized structures in the body, and so wonderful in contrivance that it is rightfully alluded to as one of the marked instances of the beneficences of God as displayed in creation.

Yet, in spite of the profundity of the researches which the ingenious mind of man has made, of late years, in the domain of science, this most important and wonderful organ has not received the amount of attention given to many other subjects.

Not only are the eyes important in themselves, but if they are strained or injured they in turn affect the general nervous system. It must be remembered that what we call "the eye" is only the eyeball; the whole optical apparatus is far more extensive than this, and is hidden away in and back of the socket, including a part of the brain itself. By means of the optic nerve the eye proper is connected with the sight-centers in the brain; and, again, the eye is nourished by the blood, which circulates to and in these parts. All treatment of the eyes must, in a certain sense, be *constitutional* (that is, general) and not local only. The latter method of treatment would be very inadequate, failing to take into account the fundamental fact that the eyes are a part of the body and dependent upon and influenced by it.

Emotions and expressions are mirrored in the eye. The "love light in the eye" has been the theme of amatory verse in all ages and times, and throughout literature we find endless references to the expression of the varying emotions of the human soul by the eyes. Passionate, burning, cruel, mystic, gentle, cunning, hot, cold, etc., are among the adjectives applied to them. The character is depicted by the eye more plainly, perhaps, than by any other organ of the body, courage, dignity and power being expressed by the organs of vision when other external indications of these attributes are lacking.

Yet, though these varying emotions and expressions can doubtless be read in the eyes, it is extremely difficult to say just *how* and *why* the eyes betray and portray them.

Some authors are of the opinion that the eye itself never changes, but only the muscles directly around it. "These muscles vary the expression," and the theory seems to be more or less borne out by the fact that, in many cases, if the parts adjacent to the eyes be covered up, no change of expression can be detected. Other authors, on the contrary, contend that the eye itself changes in expression and have advanced arguments which seem to prove it. This is an interesting line of inquiry which the student might follow for himself with interest and profit.

The eye, to be beautiful, must be clear. It must be free from defects, such as squint or dullness; the lashes must be of the proper length, the lids healthy and the whites free from the discolorations of impure blood. A perfect digestion, a healthy and energetic circulation of the blood, a delicate nervous poise, are all physical prerequisites to beautiful eyes. Form, color and size avail nothing without the luster and brilliancy of expression imparted by general physical health and tone, and though the shape and color of the eyes can never be changed, they can be greatly improved in appearance by the rational system of constitutional and hygienic treatment to be considered later.

The unfortunate tendency of modern medical science is to specialize too much; and under the influence of this tendency, general conditions are often ignored. In the majority of cases the eye specialists are no exception to this rule. They are too often inclined to treat the eye along purely local lines, instead of recognizing that it is a part of the general nervous system and treating it also along constitutional lines. Effects have been treated instead of causes; yet is is plain that the causes must be removed if we are ever to cure the effects.

The prevalence of defective eyesight is indeed alarming, did we but realize it. It has been estimated that from 25 to 50 per cent of the inhabitants of the United States are more or less short-sighted—to cite this one defect alone. At the lowest possible estimate, therefore, *at least* 25,000,000 people in this country suffer from myopia, and probably a good many more than this! And if, to this, we add those suffering from hypermetropia (or far-sight), presbyopia (old-age sight), astigmatism, squint, color-blindness and other defects of vision, we are surely safe in saying that the great majority of the inhabitants of America are afflicted with imperfect vision, and all the ills that follow in consequence.

CHAPTER II:
The Anatomy of the Human Eye ▲

A simplified exposition of the structure of this wonderful organ is imperative in a course of this character in order that the pupil may understand the terms which follow, but only a very brief summary can be attempted. For a more detailed account of the structure and physiology of the eye the student is referred to larger works.

Normally, the eyeball is nearly spherical in shape, and has three *membranes*, or coats, and three *humors*. The external coat is a thin, tough membrane, which maintains the form of the ball; it is called the *sclerotic*, and forms what is known as the "white of the eye," and includes the anterior four-fifths of the outer coat; the anterior one-fifth is the *cornea*, a transparent disk joined to the sclerotic somewhat as a watch-glass is set in its case. It can be plainly seen by looking at the eye sideways.

The next coat which lies against the inner surface of the sclerotic and is very vascular, is called the *choroid*.

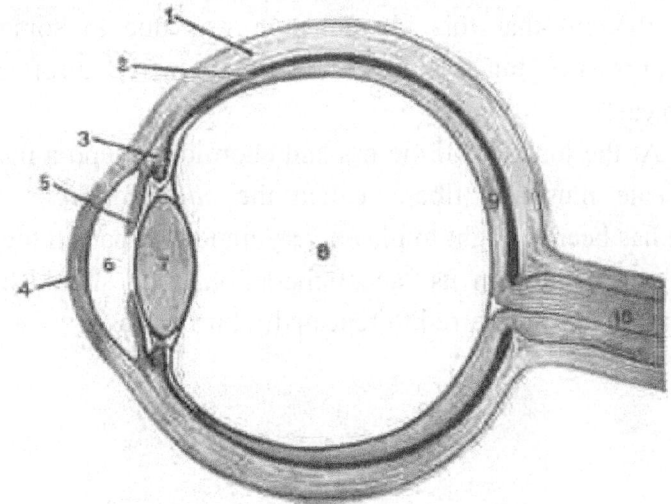

2-1. Horizontal and sectional view of the structure of the eye. (1) Sclerotic coat; (2) Choroid coat; (3) Ciliary body; (4) Cornea—the "watch glass" in front of the eyeball; (5) The iris; (6) Anterior chamber, containing aqueous humor; (7) Crystalline lens; the pupil is between 6 and 7; (8) Vitreous Humor, filling the eyeball; (9) Retina; (10) Optic nerve. ▲

The *choroid* is composed of a network of blood-vessels, and is lined with a layer of pigment cells, whose duty it is to absorb an excess of light.

The *iris*, which forms a thin curtain behind the cornea, gives the eye its special color and to a large extent its beauty. The color of the iris in newly born babies is blue, and the differing colors which come later in life are due to the addition of a greater or lesser amount of dark pigment. The color is usually more or less in uniformity with the general coloring of the individual.

The *pupil* is merely an opening in the center of the iris, and appears black because of the darkness of the interior of the eye. Through it the rays of light, coming from any object, must pass. The pupil has the power of contracting or expanding under the influence of light; and certain drugs, such as opium and belladonna, cause it to contract or dilate unnaturally for long periods of time. The pupils of cats, tigers and other animals appear to shine in the dark; and for long it was thought that this phenomenon was due to some form of phosphorescence, but it is now known to be merely a reflection from the cornea.

At the junction of the iris and choroid is found a narrow band of delicate muscular fibers, called the *ciliary muscle*. This little muscle has been thought to play a very important part in the workings of the eye, notably in its "accommodation," and should be remembered, as it will be referred to repeatedly further on.

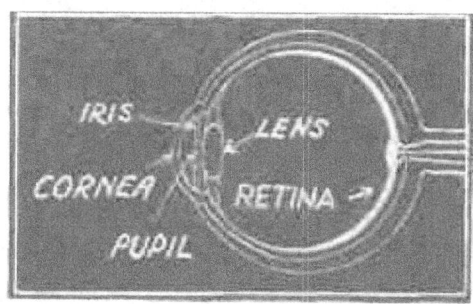

2-2. Simplified diagram, corresponding to previous image. ▲

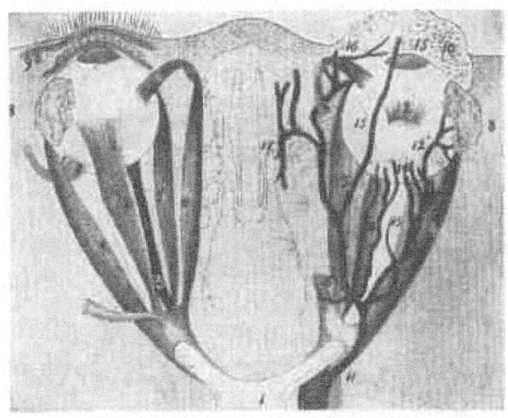

2-3. View of eyeballs from above, showing the muscles and arteries. (1) Crossing of the optic nerve; (2) Superior rectus muscle; (3) Inferior rectus muscle; (4) External rectus muscle; (5) Internal rectus muscle; (6) Superior oblique muscle (7) Inferior oblique muscle; (8) Lachrymal glands; (9) Eyelid in section; (10) Eyelid from inside; (11) Infra-orbital artery; (12) Branch to the tear gland; (13) Branch to the retina; (14) Branch to the iris; (15) Branch to the upper eyelid; (16) Branch to the eyebrow; (17) Branch to the cavity of the nose. ▲

The *retina*, the third or nervous membrane, lies at the back of the eye-wall, and upon it the light-rays entering the eye are thrown or "focused." It is an exceedingly delicate and sensitive structure, liable to injury and less than one-hundredth of an inch thick. Nevertheless about ten different layers have been found within it! The outermost of these, called "Jacob's membrane," has been found to consist of minute columns arranged side by side perpendicular to the choroid, while the internal, or nerve-fiber layer, is composed of delicate nerve-fibrils forming a surface parallel to the choroid.

The *optic nerve* passes from the eye to the brain, and carries the nervous impulses which, in the sight-centers of the brain, are converted into the "sensation of seeing." There is evidence that the optic nerve carries impulses that result in pain, but apart from this it can carry only one kind of nerve impulse, that of sight. Hence, when it is stimulated, by whatever means, whether normally by light, or by an electric current, or by a blow, we get the impression of light or "seeing stars."

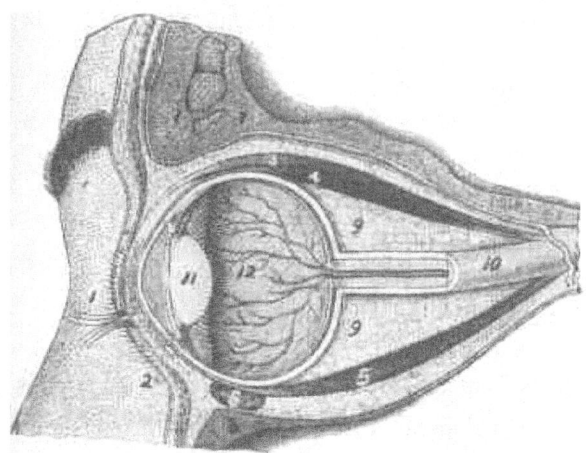

2-4. Section through the right eye. (1) Upper eyelid; (2) Lower eyelid; (3) Eyelid lifting muscle; (4) Superior rectus muscle; (5) Inferior rectus muscle; (6) Inferior oblique muscle; (7) Frontal bone; (8) Superior maxillary bone; (9) Fat; (10) Optic Nerve; (11) Crystalline lens; (12) Vitreous humor. ▲

The three humors are the *aqueous, crystalline* and *vitreous*.

The *vitreous humor* occupies about four-fifths of the interior of the ball; it is colorless and transparent, and somewhat resembles a very thin jelly. It is solid enough to maintain the shape of the eye, while at the same time yielding readily under pressure. It is firm, yet elastic.

The *crystalline humor*, or *lens*, is firmer than the vitreous, but not solid, and is shaped somewhat like an ordinary magnifying glass. It grows denser with age. This also is a very important part of the eye, and will be dealt with more fully in the discussion of accommodation and errors of refraction.

The *aqueous humor* is nearly pure water, and is contained in the space between the cornea and lens.

The orbit is the hollow cone of dense protective bone in which the eye is set. The roof of the orbit, however, is very thin, and upon this the fore-brain rests. It may be injured by a blow from beneath; and duelists are said to have selected this spot for a fatal sword-thrust.

King Henry II of France was accidentally killed at a tournament by a lance point which pierced his brain through this fragile bone.

The eyebrows are formed of bone, muscle and thick skin, covered with hairs, and protect the eyes from drops of sweat, water, dirt, etc., which might otherwise find their way into them.

The eyelid is also a protective covering, composed of a layer of loose skin, and covers the eyes during sleep, when the ball is "everted," or turned upwards, also from dust, smoke, etc.

The polish and transparency of the cornea are maintained by frequent unconscious winking, which keeps its surface moist and free from dust. The mucous lining of the eyelids is always more or less moist, and is continuous with skin at the margin of the lids. After lining the inner surface of the lids it passes over to the ball, forming a loose fold, which is the only direct connection between them; hence its name, *conjunctiva*. It covers the front part of the sclerotic, the whole of the visible portion, and lining the walls of the tear-duct, becomes continuous with the membrane of the nose and throat, and, therefore, usually takes a part in a "cold in the head," or influenza. It is usually transparent, but may become bloodshot, or yellow, as in jaundice. Yellowness results when the coloring matter of the bile is deposited in the conjunctiva.

The opening between the lids is called the *commissure*, and the apparent size of the eyes depends chiefly upon the width of this space. The almond shape of Oriental eyes is due to the unusual length of the fissure between the lids, apparently increased by the absence of the *plica semilunaris*—the small triangle of flesh at the inner angle of the eyelids. In the Chinese, the outer angle of the commissure is much higher than the inner, giving the cleft an obliquity upwards and outwards. This has a marked effect upon the whole expression of the face.

The lachrymal apparatus consists of the gland for secreting tears and the passages for draining them off. The "tear glands" are situated just above the outer angle of the eye, and a number of small ducts carry the tears, when secreted, to the eye itself. After passage across the surface of the eye, the tears are taken up by passages, which commence near the inner angle of the eye, and are conducted into the nose. The tubes carrying the tears to the nasal passages are called the *lachrymal canals*. Two tiny holes or outlets permit the tears to enter these canals from the surface of the eye. Tears are usually drained off in this manner, and only "overflow" and drop off the lids when the glands are excited by excessive emotion or by local irritation. "Sniffing" is usually the first stage of a "good cry." Infants do not shed tears before the third to fourth month, and the elephant is the only one of the lower animals accused of this human weakness—statements concerning the crocodile to the contrary notwithstanding!

The eyeball is moved in various directions by a number of muscles, attached to it at the back, top, bottom and sides. It can thus be turned upwards, downwards, inwards or outwards, or may be rotated. When these muscles are uniformly relaxed or acting in unison, the eye is normal. When, from any cause, one set of muscles exerts a stronger pull than its opposites, a squint is produced. When the muscles contract excessively, they squeeze the eyeball out of shape, elongating it or the reverse. The importance of this fact we shall see when we come to the chapter devoted to errors of refraction.

CHAPTER III:
How We See:
The Physiology and Physics of Vision ▲

The act of seeing is one of the greatest mysteries in the world. To the ancients it was an even greater mystery than to us, and continued to be so until the great astronomer Kepler noted the resemblance between the human eye and the camera, and demonstrated that images of external objects are formed by the organs of vision exactly as they are by the photographer's apparatus. In the eye, the rays of light, coming from the object seen, traverse the eyeball and fall upon the sensitive retina (the "plate" of the camera), from which they are conveyed to the sight-centers of the brain by the fibers of the optic nerve. That is, the impression which they have created upon the retina is so conveyed.

In order that the reader may understand the optics and physics of the eye, and of sight, it is necessary to say a few words concerning light, and reflecting and refracting bodies and surfaces.

Light is primarily given forth by self-luminous bodies, such as a candle or the sun; and everything else is *reflected* light. The earth reflects the rays of the sun, and this gives us our "daylight." When this reflection is cut off, dense blackness prevails. The spaces between the stars are inky black, for there is no solid body to reflect the rays coming from the sun. Rays of light are reflected when the body on which they shine sends them back. And if the light strikes a reflecting surface at an angle, the reflected angle—the so-called "angle of reflection"—is always equal to the "angle of incidence," or the direction of the shaft of light striking the object.

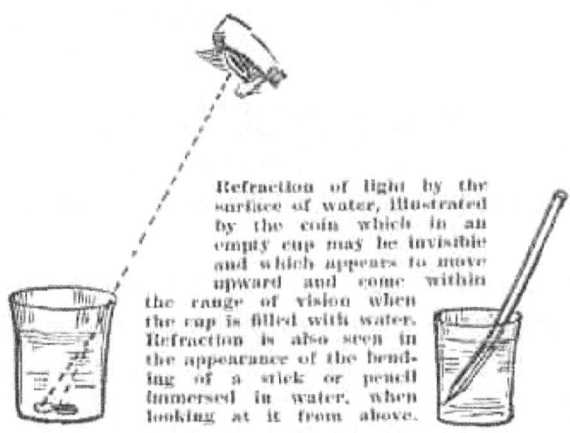

Fig. 3-1. Refraction of light by the surface of water, illustrated by the coin which in an empty cup may be invisible and which appears to move upward and come within the range of vision when the cup is filled with water. Refraction is also seen in the appearance of the bending of a stick or pencil immersed in water, when looking at it from above. ▲

The white light we see is composed, as we know, of seven primary colors. Some bodies absorb some of these vibrations, and reflect others; and when this is the case such bodies are said to be colored in various ways. The color of any object is not inherent *in* it, but is due solely to the fact that some of the light-rays are reflected and some absorbed. Those which are reflected constitute its "color."

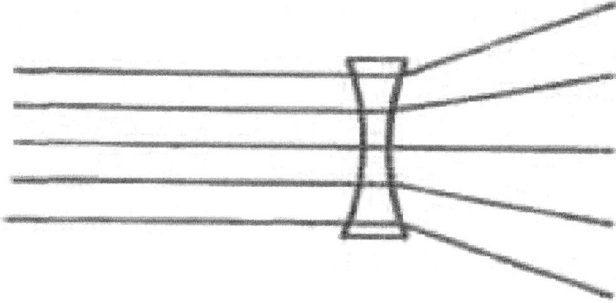

3-2. Refraction of light-rays passing through density, they concave lens, becoming divergent. ▲

When rays of light pass from one medium into another of different density, the rays are bent of their previous course, which in the case of rays coming from a distance, is one of parallel lines. A simple experiment which demonstrates this is that in which a small coin is thrown into a basin of water. It appears to be in a certain place, but if an attempt be made to touch it in this place it is found to be not there at all, but somewhere else! "Appearances are deceptive." This is due to the fact that water, being of a density different from that of air, bends the rays of light and makes them take a different direction; they are, in short, *"refracted."* By suitable means, these light-rays can be straightened out again; they may also be refracted any number of times and in various ways.

Thus, a plain, flat sheet of glass will bend all the light-rays which pass through it at the same angle. They are neither *diverged* (scattered), nor brought to a point (*converged*). When, however, the glass is double "convex," the rays of light are brought together into a *"focus."* When it is double "concave," the light-rays are scattered, or diverged.

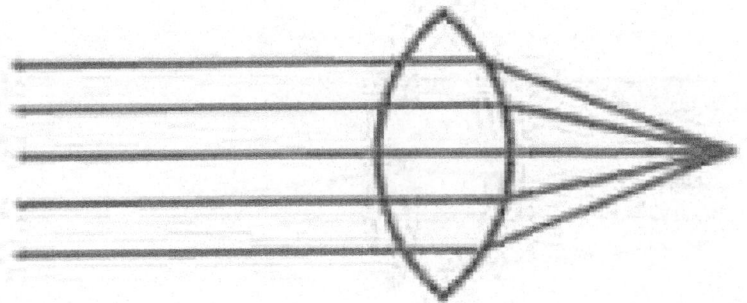

3-3. Refraction of light-rays passing through convex lens, becoming convergent. ▲

We have seen that light-rays passing through a double convex glass or lens converge at a certain point, and if, at that point, we place a screen, we catch an image of the object from which they proceed. In the eye, precisely this phenomenon takes place. The cornea and crystalline lens focus the light-rays upon the retina at the back of the eye, which catches the image, and from this point the impression is carried along the optic nerve to the brain, as before described. When the rays are focused exactly upon this delicate surface, the impression is clear and distinct. Otherwise it is blurred, or sight may fail altogether.

All parts of the retina are not equally sensitive to visual impressions. The most sensitive portion is a little depression directly in the line of vision, called the *fovea centralis*, literally, the central pit. Indeed, this is the *only* spot which admits direct vision. In all other places it is more or less blurred. We can see only one thing at a time clearly; the rest becomes blurred and fades out as it recedes from the central point. Not far from this most sensitive spot there is a *blind spot* on the retina, which is unable to see anything. We have one in each eye, but the eyes are so adjusted that when one eye is blind the other sees, and *vice versa*. This blind spot is at the entrance of the optic nerve to the retina, and its locality can easily be seen in the diagram on the preceding page.

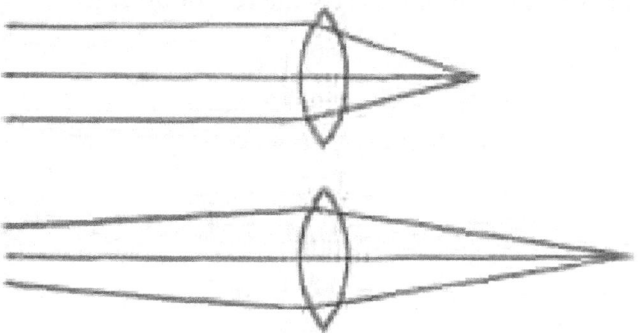

3-4. Illustrating the refraction of rays of light from distant and nearby points. The parallel rays, from a distant point, are concentrated at a point much closer to the lens than the divergent rays from a nearby point, which are focused further back. This is also demonstrated by the familiar experience of focusing light-rays in a camera. ▲

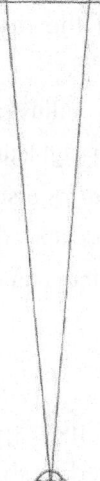

3-5. A diagram for demonstrating the "blind spot" on the retina which is the point at which the optic nerve enters. Closing the left eye and holding the diagram horizontally ten or twelve inches in front of the right eye, look fixedly upon the cross and gradually bring the diagram nearer. At from seven to nine inches the black spot will suddenly disappear from the vision because the image falls upon the "blind spot." ▲

To prove the existence of the blind spot:

Close the left eye and direct the right eye to the small cross on the left hand side of the figure. Hold the page vertically before the eye, ten or twelve inches off, and then gradually bring it nearer, still keeping the gaze fixed upon the cross. The round spot will also be visible, except at a certain distance from the eye—about seven inches—when it will disappear from view. Its image falls *upon* the point of entrance of the optic nerve, which is incapable of perceiving light.

In the diagram on this page is illustrated how the image is thrown upon the retina in the "blind spot" experiment. The eyeball in this diagram is proportionately small. The cross marks the spot of entrance of the optic nerve.

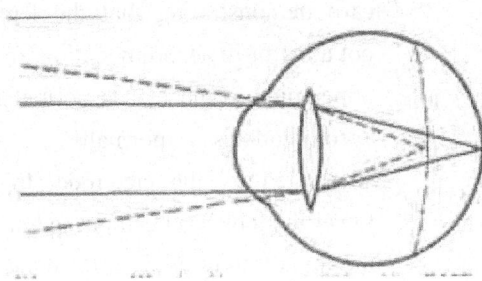

3-6. Diagram illustrating hypermetropia or far sightedness, light-rays from nearby points (indicated by broken lines) being focused behind the retina. ▲

We have seen that a double convex lens will focus light-rays at a certain point or distance beyond it; this distance will depend upon the degree of convexity of the lens. If it is only slightly convex, the focal point will be some distance away, while if it is very much curved, the focal point will be very near. We have only to alter the degree of convexity of the lens to insure the focusing of the rays at any desired distance (within limits).

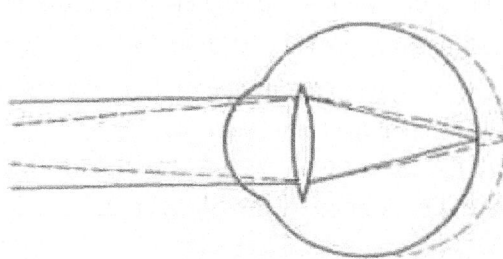

3-7. Diagram illustrating myopia or near-sightedness, rays of light from a distance (indicated by broken lines) falling in front of the retina. ▲

Now, the lens of the eye is like any other lens in this respect; and it was long ago pointed out that if it were slightly altered in shape, by means of muscular tension or otherwise, rays of light coming from different distances could be focused accurately upon the retina. It has been believed for many years that the eye adjusts itself for vision at different distances by this means, and the theory, which was accepted mainly upon the authority of Helmholtz, is the basis of the teaching in all the text books on ophthalmology today. This change of focus is called "accommodation," and is supposed to be effected by means of the ciliary muscle.

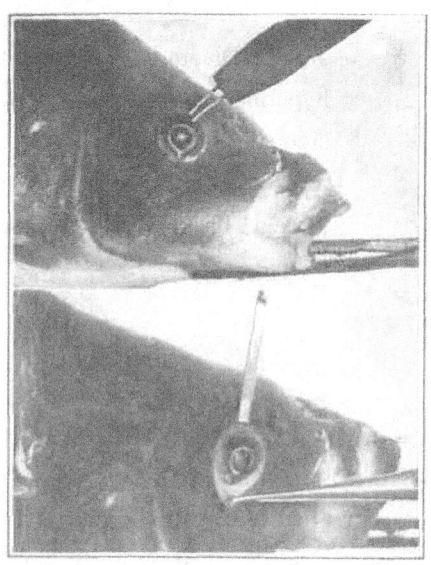

3-8. An experiment on the eye of a carp demonstrating that the lens is not a factor in accommodation. In the upper picture the eye is normal and accommodates normally when stimulated by the electrode. In the lower the lens has been pushed out of the line of sight by an instrument the point of which can be seen in the pupil. The eye is then stimulated by electricity and accommodates precisely as in the upper picture. ▲

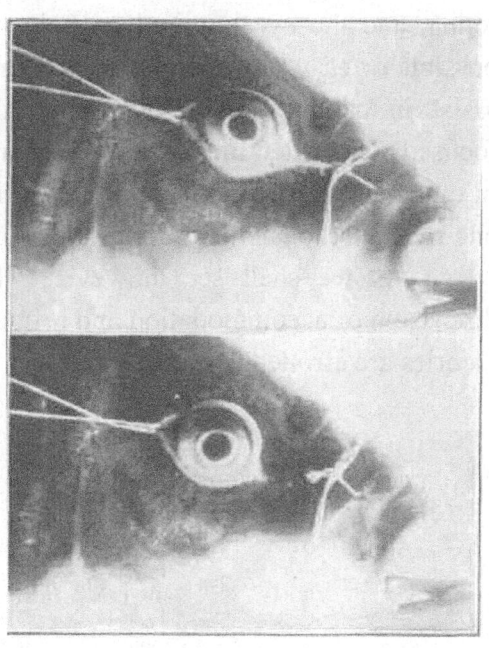

3-9. Production of astigmatism in the eye of a carp by changing the shape of the eyeball. In the upper picture the pull of two strings attached to the conjunctiva has made the cornea oval, thereby producing astigmatism. In the lower one the string has been cut, the cornea has resumed its natural shape and the eye is normal. ▲

When the eye does not adjust itself properly for vision at different distances it is said to be suffering from an *error of refraction*. These errors, with the exception of presbyopia (old-age sight), are attributed to a wrongly-shaped eyeball (occasionally to a wrongly-shaped lens), and are believed to be either congenital (present at birth) or acquired. Presbyopia is attributed to the hardening of the lens and its consequent inability to change its shape. It is stated in all the text books on ophthalmology that these conditions are incurable and almost entirely unavoidable; but, by altering the shape of the lens, the ciliary muscle is supposed to be capable of compensating to some extent for deviations from the normal in the shape of the eyeball, and when the patient is not physically at par this is believed to impose a great strain on the eye and the nervous system.

It is upon these doctrines that the treatment of refractive errors by means of glasses is based. So long as the lens and the ciliary muscle worked, and the eyeball was of the normal shape (or the lens and ciliary muscle were capable of compensating for its deficiencies), the light -rays, we have been told, were focused accurately upon the retina, and the eye required no help. But when this was no longer possible or easy, for any reason, then an extra lens was prescribed to assist in bending the light-rays so that they should be properly focused. This often improved the vision and seemed to relieve strain. In other cases it did neither, and the patient wandered hopelessly from one specialist to another in the vain search for relief.

As we shall see, however, when we come to the further discussion of accommodation and refractive errors (Chapter VI), these theories are erroneous.

CHAPTER IV:
Asthenopia: Weak Eyes ▲

Normal, healthy eyes should be strong, clear, alert and full of expression. When they are dull, weak or lacking in expression, we may be sure there is something physically or mentally wrong with their possessor Everyone has noted the meaningless expression in the eyes of the drunkard—how they roll about in a heavy, lustreless way in their sockets. This sufficiently demonstrates the intimate relationship between the eyes and the general nervous system. Indeed, it may be said that the eyes are a fair indication of the condition of the stomach and of the whole system. Excessive eating, drinking, smoking, worrying or other debilitating practices are sure to be recorded sooner or later in these delicate and sensitive structures.

When the body is normal and healthy, the blood furnished to the eyes is pure and clear. Strong eyes are the result. If, on the other hand, the digestion is out of order and the blood is impure, or loaded with unassimilated material, then the eyes grow dull and heavy; their power of vision is impaired no less than their beauty, and a wholesale degeneration of their tissues results. Eye defects of this character are almost invariably due to some constitutional weakness or defect, and not to the local causes to which they are often ascribed. This will become more apparent as we proceed. Most oculists and opticians have a tendency to treat the eye as a detached organ, without any relation at all to the rest of the body, the blood stream or the nervous structure. This is irrational, and it is impossible that any permanent good should come of it. The connection between the eye and the rest of the body is most intimate, and any form of poisoning, or weakness, in the latter at once manifests itself in the former. Under these circumstances local treatment is useless without improvement of the general physical condition. Only vigorous bodily exercise, proper diet, deep breathing and general invigoration can build up the system and place it on that high plane of energy which is essential to the health, strength and beauty of the eyes.

The causes to which the deplorable condition of civilized eyes is usually ascribed, such as prolonged use for near work, improper lighting, etc., are only injurious, as we shall see later, when the eyes are not properly used.

It usually takes a long time to tire out the eyes, and they recuperate very rapidly under proper care. Of course, if things have been allowed to go too far, a long course of treatment may be essential, but even then it is astonishing to see how rapidly recovery will take place.

Resorting to glasses as soon as any visual discomfort is experienced is a mistake—for reasons to be set forth later. The eyes are thus supplied with a crutch which partially supports them, but which, at the same time, keeps them artificially strained. The natural result is that they call for more and more powerful lenses. The proper thing to do in such cases is to find out and remove the cause of the condition, whether constitutional or local. Then all palliative* measures will become unnecessary.

*pal·li·a·tive- *adj.* 1. (of a medicine or medical care) relieving pain without dealing with the cause of the condition. *"orthodox medicines tend to be palliative rather than curative"*

CHAPTER V:
The Imperfect Sight of the Normal Eye ▲

IN the following discussion, based upon the experience of a scientist who has specialized in the field of ophthalmology, are presented facts of the greatest practical importance, not only to all those who desire to have perfect sight, but to those whose safety depends upon the sight of others. Revolutionary as these statements are, they are supported by such wealth of evidence that they cannot well be questioned.

It is generally believed that the normal eye has perfect sight all the time.

It has been compared to a perfect machine which is always in good working order. No matter what the object regarded may be, whether new, strange or familiar, whether the light is good or imperfect, whether the surroundings are pleasant or disagreeable, orthodoxy teaches that the normal eye is *always* normal and its sight *always* perfect. Even under conditions of nerve strain and bodily disease, the normal eye is expected to have perfect sight always.

This idea is very far from the truth. A careful study of the refraction of the eye extending over a period of many years has proven that no eye has perfect sight continuously. It is unusual, in fact, to find persons who can maintain perfect sight longer than a few minutes, even under the most favorable conditions. Of twenty thousand school children more than half had normal sight, but not one had perfect sight in each eye every day. The sight of many of them might be good in the morning and imperfect in the afternoon, while many with imperfect sight in the morning would have perfect sight in the afternoon.

Many children could read some letters of the alphabet perfectly, but were unable to distinguish others of the same size under similar conditions.

The degree of the imperfect sight varied within wide limits from one-third of the normal to one-tenth or less; duration was also variable. Under some conditions the imperfect sight might continue for only a few minutes or less. Under other conditions, however, a small number of students (sometimes all with normal eyes) would have sufficient loss of sight to prevent them from seeing writing on the blackboard for days, weeks, or even longer.

The sight of adults of all ages varies in a similar manner. Persons over seventy years of age with normal eyes have had attacks of loss of sight variable in degree and duration. A man aged eighty with normal eyes had periods of imperfect sight which would last from a few minutes to several hours or longer.

Both adults and children with normal eyes may have attacks of color blindness, and all persons, when their sight for form is lowered, are less able to distinguish colors than at other times. One patient, with normal eyes, perfect sight and perfect color perception in the daytime, had always been color-blind at night; he had no perception of colors after sunset.

There can be no doubt that accidents on railroads, at sea and on the streets often occur because the normal eyes of the responsible persons, *for a time*, had imperfect sight.

Unfamiliar objects almost always produce eye strain and are imperfectly seen. School children with normal eyes who can read small letters one-quarter of an inch high, at a distance of ten feet, always have trouble in reading strange writing on the blackboard, although the letters may be as much as two inches high. Strange maps always produce imperfect sight in the normal eyes of school children because they cause a strain to see. Temporary myopia, or myopic astigmatism, is always produced under these conditions, and if the strain is frequently repeated it may become continuous.

The strain may be conscious or unconscious, and may or may not produce pain, discomfort or fatigue.

Unfamiliar objects seen at the near-points are also a cause of eye strain. For this reason school children or adults learning to read, write, draw, or sew, suffer from defective vision, although they have normal eyes. In such cases temporary hypermetropia, or hypermetropic astigmatism, is produced, and with frequent repetition of the strain it becomes permanent.

This matter is of such great practical importance in the education of children that the attention of teachers should be called to the facts.*

Many children lose interest in their school work and become truants and incorrigibles from this one cause.

Light has a very important effect on vision of the normal eye; an unexpected strong light always produces defective vision. The vision of all persons is imperfect when the eyes are first exposed to the strong light of the sun, or to any strong artificial light. Rapid or sudden changes in the intensity of the light always produce defective vision, not sufficiently great to be manifest to the individual, but always to be demonstrated by careful test of the vision and by use of the retinoscope. The defective vision produced by strong light may be temporary, but it has been observed to continue in many cases for a number of weeks, frequently running into months, although it is never, probably, a permanent disability. If the eyes are gradually accustomed to strong lights, however, they will be benefited, and one may even become able to look directly at the strong light of the sun without any loss of vision whatever.

Noise is a frequent cause of defective vision in the normal eye. All persons see imperfectly when they hear any unexpected loud sound. Familiar noises do not usually lower the visual power, but unfamiliar, new or strange noises, which cause shock, always do, with the production of a temporary error of refraction. Country children from quiet schools, after they move to a noisy city, often suffer from defective vision for long periods of time. In the classroom they rarely

---

* See New York Medical Journal, Aug 30, 1913, Myopia Prevention by Teachers.

do well with their work because of impaired sight. It is a gross injustice for teachers and others to criticize, scold or humiliate such children.

The reading of small distant familiar letters, for a few minutes at least every day, is very successful in preventing these fluctuations of sight, as it tends to prevent strain in looking at unfamiliar objects. Not only the Snellen eye chart, but a calendar, a sign with small letters, or even a single small letter, may be used for such practice. The good results of this simple system of eye training justify its use in schools, in the Army and Navy, in the Merchant Marine and on railroads, as well as by every one who desires or needs continuous perfect sight.

CHAPTER VI:
Errors of Refraction: Their Cause ▲

In the two chapters following are presented the results of over thirty years of labor upon the part of a physician of high scientific standing. Until he discovered that errors of refraction were merely functional derangements, it was universally believed that they were incurable. His experiments have proved beyond the possibility of doubt that these conditions are due to the abnormal action of the muscles and that their cure is therefore a mere matter of muscular control. The details of these experiments may be found in the New York Medical Journal, May 8, 1915.

Errors of refraction are responsible for most cases of defective vision and often lead to actual disease of the eye. These errors fall into four classes: Myopia, Hypermetropia, Astigmatism and Presbyopia.

In *myopia*, commonly called short-sight or near-sight, rays of light coming from a distance are focused in *front* of the retina.

In *hypermetropia* they are focused *behind* the retina. This condition is usually called long-sight or far-sight; but in reality the sight is defective both for near and for distant vision.

In *astigmatism* the rays are not brought to a single focus, because the curvature of the refracting surfaces is greater along certain meridians than along others. There are six different kinds of astigmatism.

When one meridian is correct and the one at right angles to it myopic or hypermetropic, the condition is called simple myopic or hypermetropic astigmatism; when both meridians are hypermetropic or myopic, but one more so than the other, we get compound hypermetropic or myopic astigmatism; while a combination of myopia and hypermetropia is known as mixed astigmatism. Simple hypermetropia or myopia, without any astigmatism, is rare.

Presbyopia is that condition of the eyes which comes on usually between forty and fifty, and compels the subject to wear glasses for reading or sewing, the vision at the distance being at first apparently unaffected.

As already stated these conditions are generally supposed to be both incurable and largely unavoidable; but abundant evidence is available to show that they are purely functional troubles, and therefore both curable and preventable.

It can be and has been demonstrated, both clinically and by means of experiments on the eyes of rabbits, fish and other animals, that the lens and ciliary muscle have nothing to do with accommodation; and that, on the contrary, the shape of the whole eyeball is changed when the focus is changed, through the agency of the external muscles. When the lens have been removed from the eyes of experimental animals, or pushed out of the line of vision (as on p. 28 & 29, Chapter III), they have continued to accommodate just as before. So long as certain muscles, known as the obliques, were intact, electrical stimulation of the eyeball, or of the nerves of accommodation, always produced accommodation, but when one of them was cut accommodation could not be produced. When the severed muscle was sewed together again, however, accommodation took place as before.

These observations are in harmony with records of accommodation in the lensless human eye which may be found scattered through the literature of the subject for over a hundred years. Many persons, unfortunately, lose their lenses through the operation for cataract, and usually they are supplied afterward with two sets of glasses, one for reading, and one for distance; but occasionally such a person is able to see at both distances without any change of glasses. The correctness of these observations used to be disputed but it is no longer possible to do so, and in consequence the idea that the lens cannot be the only agent of accommodation is creeping into the orthodox literature.

From these facts it would appear that whatever may be the cause of that failure of sight which comes to most people living under civilized conditions during their later years, it cannot be the hardening of the lens; and since the change of focus in the eye depends upon the action of the external muscles, we would naturally expect that failure to focus properly would be due to failure in the action of these muscles. The accuracy of this conclusion has been demonstrated by numerous experiments upon the eye muscles of animals.

These muscles form an almost complete band around the eyeball and lengthen it when they contract, as the camera is lengthened to take pictures at the near-point.

In these experiments myopia was produced by operations increasing the pull of the obliques, leading to a lengthening of the eyeball; hypermetropia by increasing the pull of a set of muscles known as the recti, thereby shortening the eyeball; and astigmatism by operations causing an unsymmetrical change in the shape of the eyeball (as on page 28, Chapter III). Cutting one or more of the obliques, moreover, prevented the production of myopia, while hypermetropia was prevented by the cutting of one or more of the recti.

These observations leave no room for doubt that when errors of refraction exist in any eye it is because the outside muscles are squeezing it out of shape, making it, for the time being, too long or too short, or lengthening it or shortening it unevenly. Myopia is evidently due to an abnormal contraction of the oblique muscles, hypermetropia to the abnormal contraction of the recti, and astigmatism to the unequal contraction of these two sets of muscles, causing a greater elongation or shortening in one part than in another. In presbyopia the abnormal action of the recti is evidently confined at first to those periods during which the subject is looking at near objects, leaving the distant vision but slightly affected, but later on the distant vision fails also.

That these conditions cannot be due to any permanent change in the shape of the eyeball is further proven by the fact that they can be produced at will in a moment of time, as demonstrated by the retinoscope, and that they have been cured in thousands of cases, while they often disappear without treatment.

The cause of this abnormal action of the muscles is a strain, conscious or unconscious, to see, and as such is both preventable and curable.

The underlying causes of this strain are, obviously, those factors which have marked the change from primitive savage life to ultra-civilization. Improper dietetic habits, bad air and shallow breathing, insufficient exercise, too little bathing and sunlight, constipation, the excessive use of stimulants, city noises, hurry, worry, rivalry—all the physical and mental abuses ordinarily associated with civilized life—result in tension and strain of the whole body, including the eyes. Hearing and the other senses suffer as the sight does.

Of course some of the evils of civilization can not be completely overcome. The average man is likely to succumb to the powerful combination of its adverse influences if he follows the line of least resistance and makes no effort to rise above the example of his associates. But a person of average intelligence, if he understands the problem that confronts him, can, as a rule, live in the most congested centers of civilization with very little or no detriment to his health and sense organs.

CHAPTER VII:
Errors of Refraction: Their Cure ▲

In the chapter on "The Imperfect Sight of the Normal Eye" it was seen that no refractive condition is ever continuous. Eyes with ordinarily normal sight may suffer from errors of refraction at times, and eyes which are ordinarily near-sighted or far-sighted or astigmatic, may become less so, or even normal. It is obvious that this must be so, from the fact that the refraction is controlled by muscular action. But glasses cannot change as the eyes change, and therefore the mind, which wants to see, and which has a great capacity for adapting itself to adverse conditions, tries to maintain continuously the refractive condition they are designed to correct. That this tires the eyes is the experience of everyone who has worn glasses; that it must make the condition worse is obvious; and that it must be particularly harmful during the plastic years of childhood goes without saying.

The thing to do if one has an error of refraction, therefore, is not to wear glasses but to learn how to use the eyes correctly. This means seeing best with the center of sight, the fovea centralis previously alluded to, and this means that a very small part of everything one looks at is seen best and everything else less distinctly in proportion as it is removed from the central point. This is called *Central Fixation* and is the basis of the treatment of errors of refraction without glasses. When the eye looks at objects with central fixation it is at rest, the muscles which control the refraction act normally, and maximum vision is attained.

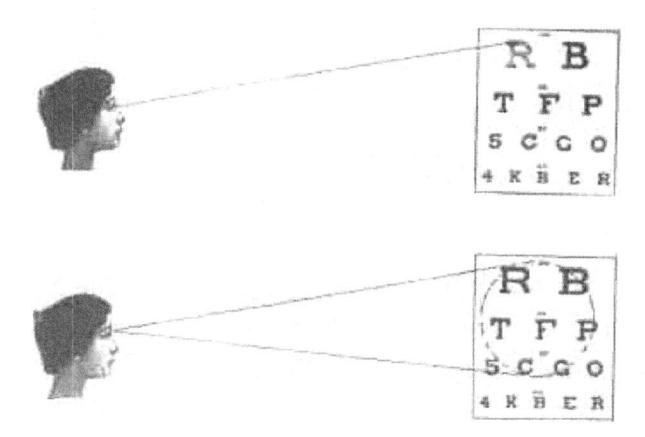

7-1. In the upper picture the sight is centered upon one spot, the upper left-hand corner of the letter R, which is seen more clearly and appears to be blacker than the rest of the field of vision. This is central fixation. In the lower picture the subject is endeavoring to see every part of her field of vision equally well at the same time. This is eccentric fixation and always accompanies eye strain. ▲

It is impossible, however, for the eye to look at any point for more than a fraction of a second. If it tries to do so, the point disappears and the whole visual field blurs. Perfect vision is thus seen to depend on clear vision of the smallest possible area and constant movement of the eye from one such area to another.

Central fixation is opposed to *Eccentric Fixation*, in which the eye partially or completely suppresses the vision of the center of the retina and sees a considerable area all alike at one time, or even sees the outer part of the visual field better than the center. In such cases not only is the central point seen less distinctly than it normally should be, but the outer parts of the field are less distinct than when the center is seen best. Black letters appear less black, white letters upon a black ground less white, and colored letters of a lighter shade than they normally would. The outlines of the letter are not clear, the margins being shadowy. Their size is altered and they appear larger or smaller than with normal vision. Their shape is distorted, and a square letter may seem to be round. Illustrations of various kinds occur, and multiple vision is common. Pain, fatigue, or discomfort of some sort is usually felt, and headaches are frequently produced.

A common symptom, also, is twitching of the eyeballs or eyelids. This is usually unconscious, but may be felt if the patient lightly touches the closed eyelid of one eye while the other is looking at a letter by eccentric fixation. The appearance of the eye is usually expressive of effort, and a greater or less degree of squint is always present. Even redness of the margins of the lids and dark circles under the eyes may be produced by eccentric fixation.

Most people whose vision is not markedly defective can demonstrate the facts of central fixation for themselves. Let such a person try to see two printed words, or even two letters, equally well at the same time. At first he will probably find himself looking from one word or letter to another, and if he really tries to see both at the same time he will find it so difficult that he may give it up before anything happens. If he is able to keep up the strain for a very brief period, however, the words will blur and become indistinguishable. If he is able to look at a small letter, however, and see it better than the others in its neighborhood, or look at one side of the letter and see it better than the other he will experience a feeling of rest.

Eccentric fixation is a symptom of strain (in which the whole body participates). The first thing for the patient who wants to improve his vision to do, therefore, is to relax this strain. One of the best ways to do this is to close the eyes, cover them with the palms of the hands in such a way as to exclude all the light, while avoiding pressure on the eyeballs (see illustration), and think of something that will keep the mind at rest. Many people like to remember something black, but any other color will do just as well if one prefers it. It is necessary to shift the attention from one part of the remembered object to another, because, as any psychologist knows, it is impossible to be continuously conscious of an unchanging object, and if one tries it he will only increase the strain. With practice it becomes easier to think of very small objects, like a period, or a very small letter, but in the beginning most people prefer something fairly large. One can also for a change think of other things, but the memory of a small object of vision seems to produce the best results.

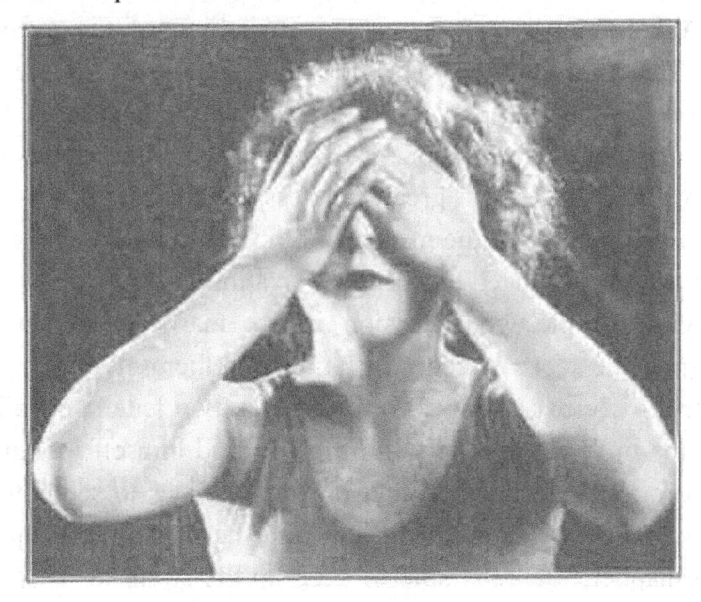

7-2. How palming is done for relaxing the strain on the eyes. ▲

If one succeeds in obtaining perfect relaxation in this way the entire visual field will become black, apart from any memory image one may have formed, because, as explained in Chapter II, the optic nerve cannot carry any sensation but that of light (unless it be the sensation of pain). If no light enters the eye, and the visual mechanism is perfectly at rest, one sees nothing —that is, black. If it is not at rest, however, one will continue to see lights and colors even without the stimulus of light. As a rule the colors are grays and browns, but in some cases they are kaleidoscopic in character. It is best, however, not to think very much about the nature of one's visual field, because as soon as he begins to do so he is liable to begin to strain. An approximate black indicates a satisfactory degree of relaxation, and most people attain it with very little trouble.

These periods of rest may be as long and as frequent as time and inclination permit. A few minutes will help, but a half-hour period, two or three or more times a day, is usually necessary for adults. Some people are more greatly benefited by an hour, or even several hours; but it is useless to attempt these long periods unless one can do it without becoming mentally worried or physically restless. In that case they become periods of strain, not periods of rest. The ability to relax in this way grows with practice.

After the eyes have been rested by palming, or by simply closing them, one should look at the letters of the Snellen test card, or at a bit of reading matter which one could not see before, and almost invariably he will find that his sight has improved, sometimes only slightly, sometimes to an astonishing degree. Occasionally this improvement is permanent, but usually it lasts for a moment only. This is the germ of improved vision from which the full flower of normal sight must grow. As soon as the strain returns, and the vision begins to lapse to its old condition, one should rest again for as long a time as is found necessary, and proceed as before. If one keeps up the practice, the flashes of improved vision come oftener and stay longer until at last they become permanent. In reading the letters on the test card one should, of course, never stare at them. If one does not see a letter, he should immediately look away, close the eyes, or palm. If one does see it, and wants to go on looking at it, he can shift from one side of it to the other.

Between periods of regular practice one can rest by closing the eyes for a moment or longer, as occasion permits, with or without the memory of a period or other small object, and sometimes one has an opportunity to palm with one hand. And one can practice on the letters of advertisements and signs, or on any small objects in one's line of vision. Some people think they are benefited by carrying about with them continually the memory of a period or small letter, but others find it a strain to remember such an object with the eyes open.

Another way to obtain central fixation is to notice that one sees a *part* of everything he looks at best, and the rest of it less distinctly in proportion as it is removed from the central point. The Snellen test card is useful for this practice. One can begin by looking from one end of a line to another, noting that he sees each best alternately. Then he can look from one letter to another and finally he may become able to look from one side to another of the smallest letters at a distance of ten or more feet and see each side best alternately.

A good way to practice at the near-point is to make a dot of about the size of a pica-type* period, and after finding the distance at which it is seen best, try, by the methods given above, to bring it out with equal clearness at greater and lesser distances. By daily practice it should become possible to see it clearly as close as three inches and as far away as twenty. Or one may do the same thing with diamond type.

* This book is printed in pica type. [equivalent to 10pt font; 10 characters per in]

When the eyes are different it is best to begin practicing both together. Later, if it is found necessary, the eye farthest from normal can be practiced separately and to a greater extent.

> Diamond type is condemned by most Ophthalmologists and Optometrists as being too fine for any eye except under most favorable conditions. My experience has been that considerable benefit can be derived from reading this because it practically necessitates central fixation. It cannot be read except when the eye is relaxed.
>
> Many Bibles and Testaments are printed in Pearl type. This small print is considered by some to be responsible for much eye weakness, but we can prove that the eye defects are the results of other causes than the small print.
>
> *It is claimed by the secretary of one of the State Boards of Health that an attempt of a boy to read a Bible printed in Agate type caused the eyes to be so weakened that school work was abandoned for two years I claim other causes were instrumental in producing this eye weakness.*
>
> Nonpareil is used for some papers and children's magazines, but is condemned by those who have a wrong idea of the use and abuse of the eyes.
>
> It is claimed that Minion may be safely used by adult or young eyes, though it is, erroneously, considered injurious for children.
>
> Brevier is frequently seen in newspapers. This should be a satisfactory type for anyone.
>
> Bourgeois is a favorite type for magazines and is very similar to Brevier.

Editor's Note:: This text box offers approximations of the original typewriter faces.

And in all cases it should be kept constantly in mind that the sight cannot be improved by effort. Strain cannot be relieved by effort, but only by "letting go."

In addition to the foregoing practices everything possible should be done to relax the mind and the whole body. It is well to begin the day with general bodily exercises. A warm or tepid sponge bath, followed by a cool or cold sponging and brisk rubbing with a rough towel, will help to maintain normal skin action. A cool eye bath, gradually growing a little cooler, but never cold enough to be uncomfortable, is an excellent local treatment for the eyes. One should take whatever measures are necessary to secure normal action of the bowels. A daily walk as long as time and strength permit, introducing short runs at intervals, will prove a great benefit unless there is some contraindication in the way of serious disease. Increased vitality is needed for health of body and eyes, and it cannot be obtained without exercise, taken in gradually increasing doses. One should breathe fresh air all night and every hour possible during the day. One should obtain sufficient sleep if one hopes to have normal eyes.

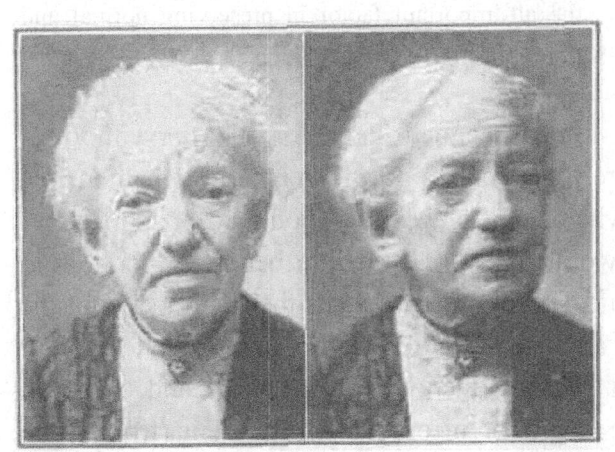

7-3. In the picture at the left the subject is looking at a Snellen test card with normal vision. At the right she is trying to see a picture at twenty feet, and the strain has produced compound myopic astigmatism. ▲

These measures are usually successful in curing myopia, hypermetropia, astigmatism and presbyopia. Patients with presbyopia, combined with other errors of refraction, and even incipient cataract, have been cured at sixty, seventy and even eighty years of age. Persons with high degrees of myopia have been cured by practicing only a few of the directions presented here. It is not necessary to understand the anatomy and physiology of the eye—however interesting and useful it may be to know these things —to be cured of errors of refraction. All that is necessary is to follow, literally and persistently, the simple directions given, every day for a sufficient length of time.

Glasses should be discarded if possible. Some people are able to make progress in spite of wearing them part of the time, but they are always a great handicap, undoing, to a greater or less degree, what has been gained by practice. If worn without change after the refraction has changed, they may also cause great discomfort.

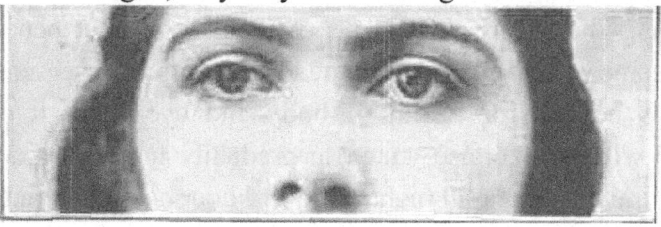

7-4. Seeing without strain, the all-important factor in preserving normal and healthy sight. This is possible only through central fixation. ▲

If the methods recommended later for the prevention of myopia in schools were practiced by people generally, whether they are old or young, or whether their eyes are good, bad or indifferent, that one thing alone would be of inestimable benefit. If any child under twelve who has never worn glasses reads the small letters of the Snellen test card, or any small letter, every day, or letters, at a distance of ten feet or more, with both eyes together and each eye separately, he will be cured of errors of refraction in from three months to two years, without any supervision or any other treatment. Adults of all ages will also be benefited by this practice, and may be cured, if they are sufficiently persistent. By such practice both children and adults will usually discover for themselves the facts about central fixation, strain, and other fundamental truths about the eyes. The time required for a cure varies greatly in different cases. Some persons are relieved immediately. In other cases weeks, months and even years of training are required. The practice should always be continued for a few minutes daily to avoid relapses. Even the normal eye requires practice in normal vision to avoid falling into errors of refraction.

CHAPTER VIII:
Amblyopia ▲

Most physicians at the present time believe that amblyopia is incurable, but it has been proved that it can be successfully treated by means of new methods of eye training. During the last ten years numerous patients, ranging in age from six to seventy-five years, have secured normal vision by this means. The facts were first reported in La Clinique Opthalmologique, December, 1912.

AMBLYOPIA is a term applied to a condition of the eyesight in which there is a lowering of visual power which can not be relieved by glasses and is not dependent on any visible changes in the organ of vision. It has been facetiously defined as a condition in which neither the patient nor the doctor can see. The patient suffers from poor vision, while the doctor can find nothing wrong with his eyes. The condition usually affects only one eye, and is so often associated with squint that it has been erroneously supposed to be both the cause and the effect of that condition.

The text books enumerate many different types of amblyopia. The one known as amblyopia exanopsia was so named because it was supposed to result from a suppression of the sight of the affected eye during early youth, owing to some defect, such as a squint or error of refraction. Such defects were supposed to prevent the retina from attaining the functional capacity of normal eyes, and the literature of the subject is full of the impossibility of cure. "The function of the retina never again becomes perfectly normal," says Fuchs, "even when the cause of the trouble has been removed."

There are, nevertheless, many cases of spontaneous cures on record, usually occurring when the perfect eye has been lost by accident. In such cases the amblyopic eye in the course of time frequently becomes normal.

It is gratifying to be able to state that the ailment is purely functional, and the authorities are quite wrong in supposing that it can not be cured. All cases have been relieved by eye training, and complete cures have been effected when the exercises were faithfully practiced. The progress has sometimes been very rapid; sight occasionally improving in a few minutes from one-fiftieth of normal to one-tenth.

In order that patients may understand the condition, they are taught how to produce amblyopia in the better eye and to increase it in the amblyopic eye by improper efforts to see. After they have learned to lower their vision voluntarily they become better able to improve it. The following case illustrates: A girl of fifteen had had amblyopia and squint since childhood. The vision of the right eye was 1/40 (of normal), while that of the left was 2/3. Glasses did not improve either eye. The patient was seated twenty feet from a Snellen test card and the right or poorer eye was covered with an opaque screen. She was then directed to look with her better eye at the large letter on the card and to note its clearness. Next she was told to look at a point three feet to one side of the card, and her attention was called to the fact that then she did not see the large letter so well. The point of fixation was brought closer and closer to the letter until she appreciated the fact that her vision was lowered even when she looked only a few inches to one side of it. When she looked at a small letter she readily recognized that an eccentric fixation of less than an inch lowered the vision.

After she had learned to increase the amblyopia of the better eye this eye was covered, while she was taught how to lower the vision of the other or poorer eye by increasing its eccentric fixation. This was accomplished in a few minutes. She was told that the cause of her defective sight was her habit of looking at objects with a part of the retina to one side of the true center of sight. She was advised to see by looking *straight* at the letters she wished to see. In less than half an hour the vision of the left eye became normal, while the right improved from 1/40 to 1/10. The cure was complete in two weeks.

Unconscious of the fact that they were looking at objects with their eyes turned to one side, many amblyopic patients had difficulty in realizing that this was the case. When they did come to understand it, it helped them to secure central fixation, and their sight immediately improved.

CHAPTER IX:
Color Blindness ▲

Both because of its scientific interest and its practical bearings, this curious defect of the eyes occupies a large place in ophthalmological literature. Although it must have existed for centuries, the first case on record was discovered in the practice of a Dr. Tuberville in 1684. Nearly a hundred years later an English chemist by the name of Dalton, who was color-blind himself, and could see no difference between the color of a laurel leaf and that of a stick of red sealing wax, published the first accurate description of the condition. For this reason continental scientists gave it the name of Daltonism.

Although it would seem to be obvious that a condition of color blindness must be very dangerous, when it exists in persons responsible for the lives of others on railroads and steamers, it was not until the latter part of the nineteenth century, after much agitation by the medical profession, that its practical bearings were recognized. Owing to the remarkable tendency of color blindness to conceal itself both from the subject and his associates, managers of transportation companies distrusted the scientists and could not be brought to believe that such a defect could exist in persons who had been in their employ for years without its being discovered.

Sweden was the first country to pass a law forbidding the employment of any man upon a railroad until his color vision had been tested. This action was taken as the result of the investigations of Prof. Holmgren of the University of Upsala, who discovered thirteen color-blind men among 266 railroad employees, and his book on "Color Blindness in Its Relations to Railroads and the Marine," had the effect of concentrating the attention of the world upon the subject. Today most shipping and railway companies require employees whose duties include the recognition of variously colored lights and signals to submit to a special examination for color blindness.

There are various degrees of color blindness. The condition in which no color can be recognized, and the world looks like a steel engraving, is rare, and its existence is denied by some. In cases where this total lack of color perception has been recorded, there has also been a considerable reduction of visual acuity* in other respects. Usually only one color is lost by the subject in this odd manner, but sometimes more than one. Thus the subject may be color-blind for red, for blue, for green, etc., as the case may be. The most common form is that in which red is deficient. Many theories have been advanced to account for color blindness, and it is generally supposed to be incurable, but the evidence at present available indicates that it is simply a functional trouble like errors of refraction. It has been relieved, even when of considerable degree, by the methods presented in this book. Practice should be taken to acquire this habit, even when there may be no other apparent trouble with or defect of vision.

a·cu·i·ty n. - keenness of thought, vision, or hearing. The ability to hear, see, or think accurately and clearly: The word comes from the Latin acuitas, which means sharpness.

CHAPTER X:
Strabismus: Squint ▲

In the following is presented a cure, the efficacy of which has been tested in numerous cases, for one of the most distressing and disfiguring of eye complaints. Only approximately curable by any of the means heretofore used, it has been found that squint always yields to eye training when persistently and intelligently used.

SQUINT, or strabismus, as it is called scientifically, is one of the vexed problems of ophthalmology. Many curious suggestions, both popular and scientific, have been made as to its cause. None of these theories come anywhere near to agreement, and while some seem to fit some cases, they leave many others unexplained.

The first definitely scientific theory advanced to account for squint was that it was due to an abnormality of the muscles which turn the eyeball in the socket. This theory seemed so plausible that it was almost universally accepted at one time, and an era of operations ensued, with many disastrous results.

Then Donders advanced his accommodation theory, which immediately came into vogue. This theory is based on the fact that when the eyes look at a near object there is not only a change of focus, but the visual axes, which are parallel when the object of vision is a distant one, are turned slightly inward. These two acts, accommodation and convergence, being always performed together, have become associated by hereditary habit so that it is difficult to converge without accommodation. Donders concluded, therefore, that an abnormal effort of accommodation resulted in abnormal convergence.

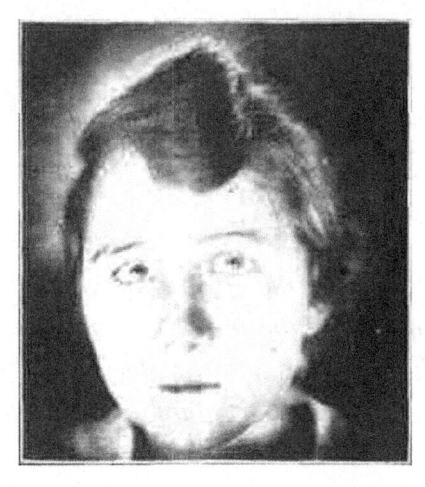

10-1. A typical case of convergent squint or "cross eyes." ▲

According to another theory, the essential or underlying cause is a congenital defect in the "fusion faculty," of the power of co-ordinating the two visual images, resulting in the development of a squint on the slightest provocation.

The truth is that squint is a purely functional defect. Some persons can produce it at will, and it is frequently produced in persons with normal eyes, both children and adults, when they try unsuccessfully to read the Snellen test card. When the eyes are not properly used, the optic axes are never parallel, although the defect is not usually sufficient to attract attention.

Squint can be cured by the same methods recommended for errors of refraction, and it is also helpful to learn how to squint voluntarily. These methods not only straighten the eye, but cure the imperfect sight which is almost invariably associated with squint. Operations, even when successful—and often they make the condition worse — are not expected to do anything more than approximately straighten the eye. They do not improve the sight.

10-2. The same patient cured by rational methods of eye training. ▲

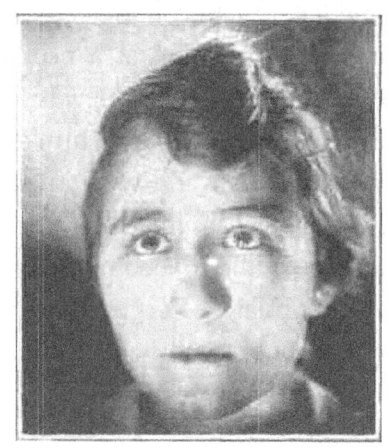

CHAPTER XI:
Saving the Sight of the Children ▲

In the following pages the first successful attempt to cure defective vision and prevent myopia in schools is described. The details may be found in the New York Medical Journal, July 29, 1911, and August 30, 1913, and are worthy of more attention than they have received. The prevention of myopia among school children is of vital and far-reaching importance. Eye defects, with the nervousness, headaches and irritability for which they are responsible, not only prevent children from availing themselves of the educational opportunities offered to them by the state, but are often a serious handicap as well as a discomfort and an expense in later life. If there is any way of preventing such tragedies it ought to be adopted without a moment's delay. Meantime parents can protect their children by using the methods advocated at home. Since it is difficult to prove a negative proposition, it cannot, of course, be absolutely proven that these methods actually prevented myopia, but since all cases of defective eyesight were improved by them there can be no reasonable doubt that they also prevented this condition.

One of the most serious problems which civilization has been called upon to solve is that of saving the sight of children. Ever since the introduction of popular education it has been recognized that the system was disastrous to the eyesight of the rising generation. Voluminous statistics, collected both in this country and in Europe, show that whereas most children on entering school have perfect sight, the percentage of eye defects steadily increases during the educational process, reaching its climax in the higher institutions of learning.

In Europe, where the military system has made the matter one of great practical importance to the State, much effort has been made to find a remedy for the evil, and millions of dollars have been spent in carrying out the suggestions of the eye specialists. The lighting of the schools, the furniture, the print in the school books, the position assumed by the pupils at work, were all regulated in accordance with expert opinion. In some cases the suggested reforms were carried out with such thoroughness that "face-rests" were attached to the desks to prevent the children from getting their eyes too near their books.

The injurious effects of the educational process were not, however, appreciably arrested. Cohn reports, indeed, an increase both in the percentage and degree of myopia in those schools in which he had especially exerted himself to secure reforms, while Just found that the excellent hygienic arrangements in the high school of Zittau, where he examined the eyes of 1,229 of the pupils, had not in any degree lessened the percentage of myopia.

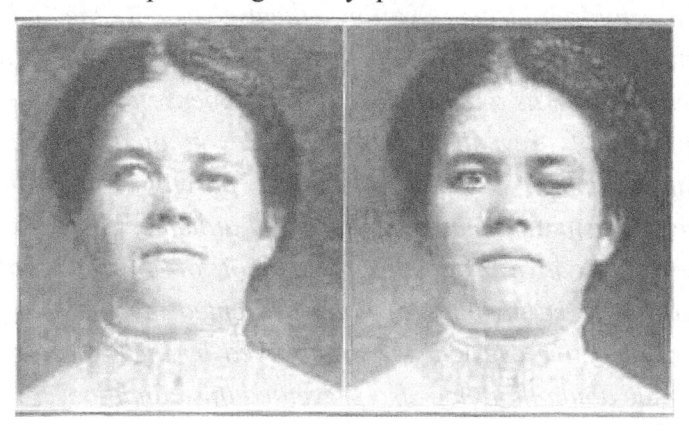

11-1. A case of divergent vertical squint ultimately cured by educational methods. In the picture at the left the right eye turns out and up, while the left eye looks straight. At the right the patient has learned to look straight with the right eye, while the left turns down and out. ▲

All these efforts to prevent myopia failed because they were based on a wrong conception of the cause of the condition. It was naturally supposed that the cause of the failure of the eye to see distant objects was its too constant use for near work; but this theory is gradually giving way before statistics, and the orthodox writers have now fallen back on that convenient scapegoat, heredity, for an explanation. Since some people are able to use their eyes continuously for near work without getting near-sighted, and others get near-sighted without any appreciable amount of such work; since the limitation of such work fails to check the progress of the trouble; and since domestic animals and wild animals in captivity, although they neither read nor sew, develop high degrees of myopia (as shown in numerous investigations);—there is obviously some other influence at work, and this influence is now supposed to be heredity.

It is known that people are rarely if ever born myopic, but they are supposed to be born with a tendency to that condition, and near work is generally believed to accentuate this tendency. As there is no way of finding out who has this unfortunate bent and who has not, the old precautions are, therefore, still insisted upon for the most part, although some authorities attach very little if any importance to them, maintaining that when one has the myopic tendency one might as well resign oneself to one's fate and not bother with tiresome precautions.

As a matter of fact the retinoscope has demonstrated that straining to see at the near-point never produces myopia, but, on the contrary, hypermetropia, as already noted in Chapter V, on "The Imperfect Sight of the Normal Eye." Myopia is produced by straining to see distant objects, and it has been found that it is produced whenever children with normal vision strain to see unfamiliar distant objects. (See also Chapter V.)

When regarding familiar distant objects it is quite otherwise. Daily exercise in the distant vision of familiar objects, therefore, suggests itself as the best method of preventing the tendency to strain in viewing unfamiliar distant objects and thus of preventing permanent myopia and hypermetropia. This method has been tried in many public schools during the last fifteen years and has been uniformly successful, not only in preventing myopia, but in curing it where it already existed.

The Snellen test card was found to be the best distant object for exercises in distant vision. When memorized it becomes a familiar distant object. Its daily use for half a minute or longer both prevented and cured myopia, and also improved the vision for near objects, many pupils stating that they were able, after its introduction into the classroom, to study with less or no discomfort. The test card was placed permanently where all the pupils could see it from their seats, and the children were instructed by the teachers to read it daily with both eyes together and with each eye, separately, the other being covered with the palm of the hand in such a way as to avoid pressure on the eyeball. Records of vision were made either with the same card or with an unfamiliar one. This method of preventing myopia was used for eight years continuously in the public schools of Grand Forks, North Dakota, and reduced the percentage of myopia from six to one percent.

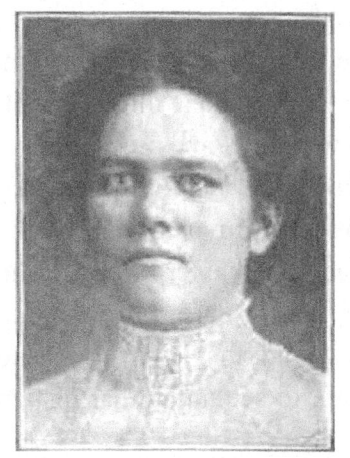

11-2. The same patient after a complete cure had been effected. All four pictures were taken within fifteen minutes of each other, the patient having learned to reproduce voluntarily the conditions represented. ▲

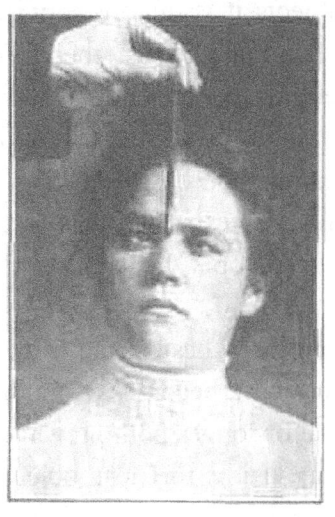

11-3. A part of the treatment. The patient has learned to turn both eyes in by looking at a pencil held over the bridge of the nose. Later she became able to turn them in without the pencil, or to turn either eye in while the other remained straight. ▲

Later it was introduced into a number of public schools in New York with a total attendance of ten thousand children. The cards were received with considerable skepticism, the teachers being unable to believe that such a simple method, and one so entirely at variance with previous teachings on the subject, could produce results. Some of the teachers neglected to use them, but others, in spite of their miscellaneous and often trying duties, gave the matter serious attention, and were able to present complete reports covering five thousand children. Of this number three thousand had defective eyesight and the reports showed that more than a third of this number gained perfect vision in both eyes after the test cards were introduced.

In one case in which there had been twenty-seven defectives in a class, twenty-five were reported cured and two much improved, while one incorrigible and one truant had become good students because, after they had obtained normal vision, they were able to study without pain or discomfort.

The Snellen test card was devised by Herman Snellen, Professor of Ophthalmology in the University of Utrecht, for the purpose of testing the sight by means of letters and figures of different sizes, but it has been found equally valuable for eye training. Each line is designated by a number indicating the distance in feet at which it should be read, but this is only a minimum standard. Many people become able to read the various lines at twice the distances marked and a few at three times these distances. The records of vision are written in the form of a fraction, the upper line (numerator) indicating the distance in feet of the reader from the card, and the lower (denominator) the line read. When the numerator and denominator are equal, the sight is normal. The school records were made as follows, the vision of each eye being recorded separately:

Subject	February 1913		April, 1913		June, 1913	
	R.	L.	R.	L.	R.	L.
John D	20/100	20/50	20/50	20/40	20/20	20/20
Sam G	20/50	27/70	20/30	20/40	20/15	20/20

That the improvement shown by the records was due to the use of the cards was demonstrated not only by the fact that when the cards were removed relapses occurred where improvement had not been sufficient to establish its permanence, but also by comparative tests made with and without cards. In one case six pupils with defective sight were examined daily for one week without the use of the test card. No improvement took place. The same six pupils were then given daily exercises in distant vision with the test card. At the end of that time they had all improved and five were cured. In the case of another lot of six defectives in the same school the results were similar. No improvement was noted during the week that the card was not used, but after a week of exercises in distant vision all had shown marked improvement, while at the end of a month all were cured.

In a considerable proportion of cases the children learned in a few minutes how to look at things without effort and were thus cured of their myopia. Many of the teachers were also cured of eye troubles and enabled to discard their glasses.

CHAPTER XII:
Common Diseases of the Eye ▲

In addition to "errors of refraction," there are certain diseases of the eye and its appendages which require special mention, since these are quite frequently met with, and their treatment is often limited, in orthodox practice, to purely local measures, neglecting the constitutional treatment which is usually so necessary, and also the measures for relief of eye strain which we are advocating.

The eye is made up, as we have seen, of numerous parts, and each of these parts may become diseased; thus we have diseases of the iris, conjunctiva, retina, eyelids, optic nerve, etc., as the case may be. We shall mention the most important of these, giving their chief causes and most effectual means of cure in each case.

CONGESTION OF THE CONJUNCTIVA

This often results, in a mild form, after exposure of the eyes to smoke, or even to strong winds. The conjunctiva is, however, nearly always inflamed in measles, and frequently in scarlet fever and smallpox. Occasionally a diphtheric membrane is formed over it, either with or without an accompanying infection of the throat. These, however, are exceptionally severe cases. In most instances, a more or less readily curable congestion results—partly from the causes mentioned, and partly from the general physical condition of the patient. If the blood is full of impurities, it aggravates the congestion. These cases are relieved from within by those hygienic and cleaning measures which tend to purify the blood stream, and carry away poisonous material.

As regards the external treatment of the eye, frequent eye baths in moderately cold salted water will be found beneficial. These may be followed by the application of cold wet cloths to the eyes, changing them as frequently as occasion may require. The patient must keep the eyes closed as much as possible.

CATARRHAL CONJUNCTIVITIS

Also referred to as "Catarrh of the Eye," results largely from a prolonged continuation of conditions similar to those which produce congestion. Those suffering from this complaint often feel as though sand were in the eyes. It is frequently met with in large cities, where dust and smoke tend to keep the eyes inflamed. The eyes are often found glued together on awakening. The mucous membrane of the eye is affected in much the same way as those of the nose and throat, and often at the same time.

Constitutional and local treatment, as advised for congestion, with complete rest for the eyes, is unquestionably about the best remedy for this trouble. When the lids are swollen and the eyes red and hot, an eye bath in salted water may be employed to advantage several times a day. If inflammation is especially severe, a weak solution of boric acid, ten grains to an ounce of water, may be employed. Poultices, eye waters and remedies of that sort should be avoided. Burning of the lids can nearly always be alleviated by an eye bath.

GRANULAR CONJUNCTIVITIS: TRACHOMA: GRANULATION OF THE EYELIDS

All these are names for the same malady, which is merely a severe form of the two former complaints. Violent inflammation of the eye, which is covered with numerous nodules, is the principal characteristic. It is a tedious and obstinate complaint, unless treated in a prompt and efficient manner. The inner surface of the lids often becomes thickened and rough, like sandpaper, and, by constant friction, impairs the transparency of the cornea. Trachoma is very contagious and in all cases precautions should be taken to avoid communicating the disease by allowing the smallest particle of the discharge from the eyes to come into contact with a healthy eye. Appropriate antiseptic treatment will be helpful. An eye-wash made from sulphate of zinc—about one grain to an ounce being the usual strength—is often effective in terminating the symptoms of this trouble, though this suggestion does not in any way eliminate the necessity for careful constitutional treatment.

PURULENT CONJUNCTIVITIS

This is often found in the newly born, and results from gonorrheal infection from the mother. It often produces blindness, unless promptly treated with nitrate of silver under proper medical supervision. This should be followed by the strictest care and cleanliness. The discharge, which is thick and yellowish, and, in bad cases, very copious, is undoubtedly and virulently contagious. Fortunately, the disease is rarely met with among adults.

STYES

These are a very painful species of small boils which form generally on the edge of the eyelids. The disease usually follows more or less the course of ordinary boils, and is nearly always brought about through constitutional causes, general debility, a disordered stomach, impure blood, etc., though eye strain is the usual immediate cause. If treatment is begun at the first sign of the appearance of the styes, they may be absorbed without suppuration, but if well started, relief may be secured more speedily by allowing them to come to a head. Hot compresses will hasten this desirable end. Usually they will open themselves when ready to discharge the pus, though in some cases it is necessary to open them with a lance. A permanent cure can be effected only by adopting constitutional treatment and learning how to use the eyes properly, thus avoiding strain. It is hardly necessary to say that strict cleanliness and adequate drainage of the parts are essential in this condition. The practice of eye relaxation and of central fixation should be observed by every one subject to styes.

DISEASES OF THE CORNEA

These are troublesome and often difficult to treat and still more difficult to diagnose properly by an unqualified practitioner. Says Dr. Black, in his work on the eyes:

"Diseases of the cornea may destroy or impair its transparency, or the ulcers that are frequently formed may extend through its substance, allow the aqueous humor to escape, and involve the iris. Even when such ulcers heal most favorably, they leave a permanent scar in the form of a white speck. Inflammation of the cornea is usually painful and accompanied by distressing sensitiveness to light. It occurs most frequently in persons whose health has been subjected to some depressing cause, or in children who have inherited a delicate constitution. Many of the latter are subject to repeated attacks for years, but the tendency to their recurrence generally disappears before adult life, and if care be taken to prevent each attack from leaving a permanent mark, the eyes may finally remain sound and strong. . . . A large, white opacity of the cornea is often mistaken for cataract, and not many years ago, when a knowledge of diseases of the eye was not so general as now, this mistake was sometimes made by physicians, and such patients were sent hundreds of miles to have the cataract removed."

It is hardly necessary to point out that, though "delicacy of constitution" might *predispose* certain person to this disease, the actual *causes* are an overloaded circulation, poor digestion, poor light, excessive use of tobacco and alcohol, etc.

This being the case, the treatment for all forms of these diseased conditions is obvious. A rigid diet, preceded, if possible, by a few days' fasting; plenty of water-drinking; eye baths; fresh air; exercises which tend to build up and strengthen the general bodily tone, etc., are all essential. Plenty of good light and sunshine are imperative at all times.

IRITIS

Also called inflammation of the iris, often destroys the sight by closing the pupil and shutting off the light from the interior of the eye. It may be accompanied by inflammation of the conjunctiva, and hence be overlooked until well developed. It should always be suspected when, in an acute affection of the eye, the sight is decidedly diminished and there is some pain in the ball, and particularly in the brow, the latter being always more severe at night. The cause is usually syphilis or rheumatism, and one of the chief aftereffects to be feared is the permanent contraction of the pupil. Local treatment is of little avail, but the application of hot and cold cloths alternately to the eye will usually assuage the pain. The patient should be careful not to use the eyes more than is absolutely necessary.

CATARACT

This is a disease of the crystalline lens, in which this body gradually loses its transparency. The pupil thus loses its natural blackness, the whitish surface of the opaque lens being seen just behind it. Cataracts are not "on the eye," as is commonly supposed, but *in* it. Until lately, it has been contended that the surgeon's knife was the only remedy, but other methods of treatment are now coming in, and it is highly probable that as soon as these newer methods become more widely known and recognized by the medical profession, operations will not be found necessary in any but advanced cases.

There are two kinds of cataracts—the old, hard cataract, and the so-called "soft" cataract. In the majority of cases the lens becomes hard and stonelike, and sight is restored by removing it, the operation having been successfully performed in many instances. In such well-advanced cases, it is probable that all the physical culturist can do is to encourage such a condition of good health that the operation can be well borne, and keep the blood as pure as possible, to carry on the good work of repair afterwards. By preserving the health, however, and using the eyes properly, cataract may be prevented; and prevention is better than cure here as elsewhere. In their earlier stage, cataracts have been permanently cured by hygienic treatment and eye education.

The reason for this is simple enough. It is this: The lens is composed of a number of transparent layers superimposed one upon another— like a number of sheets of glass laid flat one upon another. When these all lie flat and even, the light can penetrate them all equally and without interference; but if they become separated or warped, then the light-rays are bent and warped, and the otherwise transparent medium becomes more or less opaque. This is what happens in the case of cataract. By improper use of the eyes these delicate layers are disarranged. Instead of lying flat, some of them are bent or warped, preventing the free passage through them of the light-rays. If this state has been permitted to continue long enough a degenerative change within the eye takes place. When this happens, probably the only relief procurable is by removal of the lens, and thanks to the advance of modern surgery, this may now be done in the majority of cases with relative safety.

Both clinical and experimental proof that this theory is correct is forthcoming. If you take a bullock's eye, and squeeze it, you can *instantly* produce cataract—with the typical white, glassy look in the pupil. As soon as the pressure is removed, the eye again becomes normal. The little "plates" have been bent and warped, and functional cataract has been produced. This theory of cataract is also sustained by the fact that such patients actually do get well, under the influence of eye education, whereas formerly there was considered to be no help for them. All they could do was to wait, in gradually increasing blindness, until the lens was "ripe" for removal.

Constitutional causes also contribute to the production of cataract. The lens has to be nourished, like any other part of the body; but if the circulation is sluggish and the blood impure and lacking in its normal water content, the layers dry out, becoming not only less transparent, but more liable to disarrangement by the abnormal pressure of the outside muscles associated with errors of refraction.

The regime which sufferers from incipient cataract should adopt, therefore, is the following: Comply strictly with all the laws of health, including an abstemious* diet with plenty of fruit, green vegetables, and water, and no alcohol; take regular exercise and use all other methods of improving the circulation; use eye baths and similar local measures of relief; and practice daily the exercises necessary to relax the external eye muscles.

abstemious *adj.* - not self-indulgent, especially when eating and drinking.

These methods have, in many cases, either cured or greatly relieved the condition, or checked its progress, the results depending on the condition of the eye at the beginning of the treatment, the general health of the patient, his mental responsiveness, and the amount of time available for eye training. If they are adopted at the very beginning of such cases, there is every reason to believe that the majority of cataracts can be overcome in their initial stages, and before they develop to the point where they become organic.

GLAUCOMA

Glaucoma is a disease which frequently results in blindness and about which little is known. It is thought that an excess of fluids in the eye makes the ball tense and hard, and exerts injurious pressure upon its delicate contents. In acute cases, it is intensely painful, and rapidly destroys sight by pressure upon the optic nerve. In its earliest stage, its progress has been checked by the removal of a piece of the iris, or of tapping or incision through the sclerotic coat, but the operation is very uncertain in its results and sometimes seems to make the condition worse. When the optic nerve is once affected other complications arise.

In no other disease is early diagnosis and treatment more important, and many of its victims have been condemned to blindness by delay. No one with a violent pain in the eye and head, particularly if it is accompanied by flashes of light, rainbow colors and dimness of vision, should allow himself to be lulled into a sense of security by thinking it is "neuralgia."

Although the ultimate and true causes of glaucoma are as yet unknown, the thing to do, immediately it has been diagnosed, is to adopt a very abstemious diet, following a fast of a few days, if possible; use all those measures which tend to build up the general health; discard glasses if possible, and practice the various methods of eye education. Frequent cold eye baths may also be useful. In all cases a specialist should be consulted at once, if the victim has not the courage to adhere to the treatment suggested here.

DISEASES OF THE CHOROID AND RETINA

These diseases can be detected only by means of the ophthalmoscope, but may be foretold by increasing dimness of vision. They usually develop painlessly, and hence are as insidious as they are unfortunate. Long continued eye strain is one of the causes of these conditions. The excessive use of tobacco and alcohol is also, probably, an important factor; hence the necessity of giving them up completely when treatment is begun. Syphilis and kidney disease are common causes.

ATROPHY OF THE OPTIC NERVE.

This is a very serious progressive disease, resulting in total blindness. Syphilis is a frequent cause, and it goes without saying that such condition would be impossible in a healthy body, or in one wherein the seeds of disease had not been sown.

THE HEREDITARY TRANSMISSION OF EYE DISEASES

There is evidence to show that a certain number of eye diseases—or rather the *tendency* to these diseases—may be acquired by means of heredity. In color blindness this is particularly marked, as well as in certain peculiarities or conformations of the eyes. Actual *diseases* are probably not inherited, and errors of refraction are probably acquired in each generation. A tendency to gouty or rheumatic iritis, it has been contended, may be inherited; but here again it is probable that no more than the *tendency* is ever passed on in this way. A peculiar affection, "retinitis pigmentosa," which is recognized, with the ophthalmoscope, by the presence of black spots upon the retina, shows a marked tendency to hereditary transmission. It also occurs in several members of the same family, though there may be no history of it in the family. The prominent symptoms are "night blindness" and a gradually increasing contraction of the field of vision. (This is also a characteristic of certain forms of hysteria.) It is also probable that "nyctalopia," or the reverse condition—ability to see in the dark—is to some extent hereditary. But it may be laid down as a general rule that eye diseases—like all other diseases—are not hereditary, but are acquired by each generation, and by each individual for himself or herself.

EYE HEADACHES

As already mentioned, the eyes and the whole nervous system are very intimately connected; and it is well known that a constant strain upon the eyes will induce a general condition of strain, nausea, backache, etc., in addition to frequent and sometimes severe headaches. Some physicians have gone so far as to assert that true and organic diseases have been induced in this manner; but this view is no longer generally held by the medical profession. Hewetson, Noyes, Weir Mitchell and others, however, have published numerous facts showing the close connection between defective eyesight and headache, with general nervous and physical impairment of the health; and when we consider the constant strain involved, the reason for this is obvious. Some of the early symptoms are a feeling of fatigue and tension, especially above the eyes, with indistinct and confused vision in reading, writing and other close work. Following this, slight headaches will be experienced, at the base of the brain; and these will be followed or accompanied by nausea, vertigo and general nervousness. Other physical and mental symptoms may follow. When these appear, it is high time to begin treatment of the eyes.

The usual treatment in cases of this kind is a prescription for glasses; and there is no doubt that relief has often been obtained by their use.

Such measures, however, are only palliative and not ultimately curative. When the external muscles are squeezing the eyeball out of shape, glasses may correct some of the results of that condition, and by so doing may make the patient more comfortable; but they can not relieve the fundamental trouble. On the contrary, as has already been shown, they must make it worse. The only real remedy is to be found in the methods described in "Errors of Refraction: Their Cure." In the absence of such treatment glasses may prove useful, in some cases. In others they fail entirely. If it seems necessary to resort to them, and there can seldom be any legitimate excuse for such a course, they should be carefully fitted by a competent oculist and should not be worn any more than is absolutely necessary, as they serve to confirm the eyes in their bad habits. Eye headaches can often be relieved in a short time by proper hygienic methods. It is hardly necessary to say that the general health should be built up. Massage of the back of the neck and head will often bring material and instantaneous relief from the pain, and cold wet compresses to these parts will soothe and relieve the local congestion. A salt eye bath often relieves.

SYMPATHETIC INFLAMMATION

When one eye is injured by the entrance of some foreign body, or by a wound, the injury does not always limit itself to that eye. The other eye is also affected, and becomes inflamed through sympathy. This is noticeable even in slight injuries;but in grave cases it may become so serious as to necessitate the removal of the injured eye (that is, if the injured eye is so badly hurt as to render it blind and useless). In our days, this operation is not so serious as it used to be.

CHAPTER XIII:
Injuries to the Eye ▲

The eye is one of the most delicate portions of the human body; and although Nature has endeavored to protect it from injury by embedding it deep within the skull, surrounding it, so far as possible, with a circular orbit of bone, and veiling it with lids that close at the slightest hint of danger, it can not always escape injury. This chapter will treat of the most common of the accidents to which it is liable, and of the speediest and most efficient measures that can be adopted in such cases.

FOREIGN BODIES IN THE EYE. Probably the most common form of injury from which the eyes suffer is that resulting from the intrusion into it of small particles of dust, cinders, etc. These cause extreme discomfort, if not actual pain, accompanied by a flow of tears. This watering of the eye is really an effort on the part of nature to expel the offending substance, the water tending to wash the particle from the eyeball, and into the lachrymal canals, which carry it into the nose. If the particle lodges in the corner of the eye, it can be removed by means of the corner of a handkerchief, or a point twisted into it. Most foreign substances can readily be removed in this manner —provided the eye be not *rubbed*. If you rub the eye, it tends to embed the grit, or whatever it may be, more deeply in the eyeball, and if the substance has sharp points, it is liable to become so deeply embedded that it becomes difficult to remove. If, when a foreign body finds its way into the eye, the temptation to do this be resisted, the substance can readily be removed in practically every case.

Smooth bodies rarely cause much trouble, but bodies having rough cutting edges may often lodge in the conjunctiva and cause intense pain. The right method of extraction is to *evert* the eyelid*, when it will be found easy in the majority of cases to remove the cinder, or whatever it may be, by means of a small, clean, soft paint brush or the corner of a handkerchief. Direct the patient to look downwards, if the body has lodged on the upper eyelid, then turn the eyelid back over a toothpick, match or pencil. If the body is seen to be near the edge of the upper lid, it can often be removed by lifting the

*e·vert - *v.* turn (a structure or organ) outward or inside out.

lid up by means of the eyelashes, and bringing it over the lashes of the lower lid. These then act as a sort of broom, and sweep out the foreign body. As in all such cases, the free flow of tears is helpful.

When a foreign body has lodged in the firmer tissue of the cornea, its extraction is not so simple a matter, and rubbing only presses it in more firmly. In such cases, the particle is often driven in with considerable force, and it is usually so small that a magnifying glass must be employed to see it clearly. If the body be of iron or steel, it may be extracted by means of a magnet made for that purpose, otherwise a surgeon had best be sent for at once, as lasting injury may result if the substance be left in the eye too long, or if the eye be perforated, and the interior liquids allowed to escape.

WOUNDS made with pointed instruments, such as a knife, scissors, pin, etc., sometimes injure the cornea and lens, and the after-effect is frequently a cataract, when the eye is not totally lost. These, the formation of connective tissue, are usually absorbed in young people, but in older persons they may require an operation for their removal.

LIME may be splashed in the eye, and this is a dangerous form of injury. Quicklime is a powerful caustic, and often causes complete blindness by destroying the cornea. When this substance gets into the eye, it should be washed out as quickly as possible with water, and then with a solution of weak acid and water—say, a teaspoonful of vinegar to a glass of water. An equally efficient and more soothing method, however, is to bathe the injured eye in sweet oil.

In case of injury by *acids*, one part of lime-water to three of water may be used, or the eye may be freely bathed in milk. These alkalis neutralize the acid, and make it harmless or less harmful.

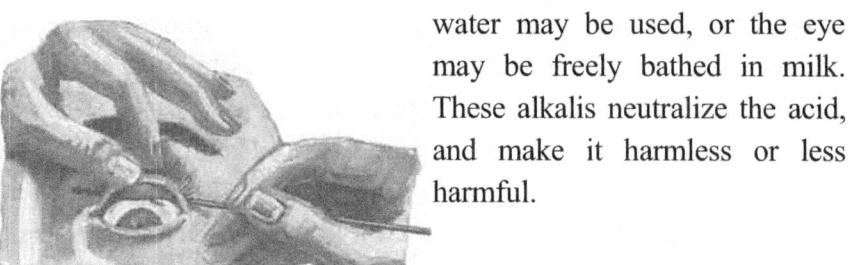

13-1. Showing the method of everting the upper eyelid for examination or removal of cinders or other foreign bodies. ▲

CHAPTER XIV:
Eye Exercises ▲

Nothing could be more evident than the fact that exercise of the eyes will strengthen these organs just as exercise of any other part of the body will strengthen that part.

Exercise of any group of muscles not only tends directly to strengthen those muscles, but it so improves the circulation as to improve the condition of the adjacent parts. If any part of the body is weak, flabby, ineffective, exercises which involve the use of the muscles in that region will have a strengthening and toning-up effect. This applies with special force to exercises for the muscles of the eye.

Most persons will be surprised, perhaps even amazed, at the improvement in the condition of the eyes, resulting from two or three weeks of proper exercise of the eye muscles. This does not mean that one should keep up this work for only two or three weeks. If you will make it a daily practice you can expect to enjoy strong eyes and good vision to perhaps the end of life.

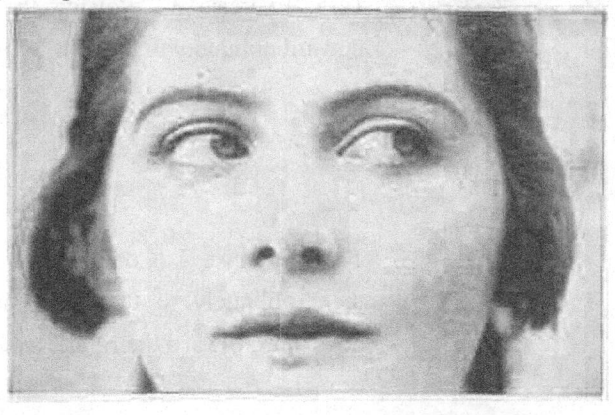

14-1. Exercise 1.—Turn and stretch the eyes far to the left ▲

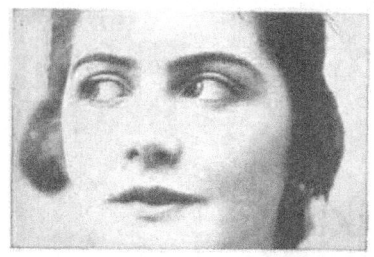

14-2. Exercise 1 (Continued).—Then turn and stretch them far to the right, continuing the movement back and forth from left to right ten times or more. ▲

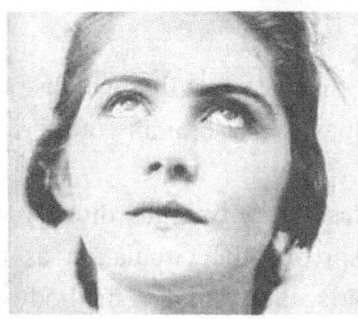

14-3. Exercise 2.—Turn the eyes upward, that is to say, look as far upward as possible without raising the head. ▲

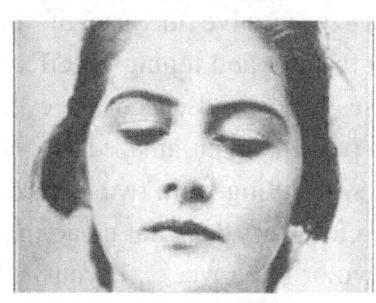

14-4. Exercise 2 (Continued).—Then, without moving the head, lower the eyes, looking as far down as possible. Continue raising and lowering the eyes ten times or more. ▲

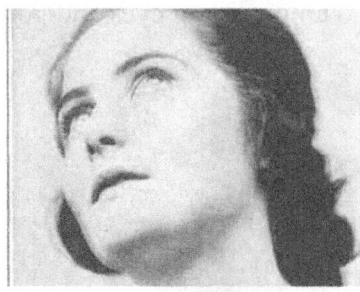

14-5. Exercise 3.—Raising the eyes, look upward obliquely to the left. ▲

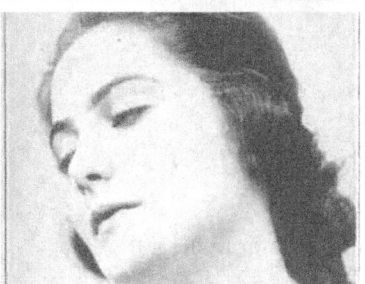

14-6. Exercise 3 (Continued).—Then lower them obliquely to the other side, looking downward toward the right. Repeat ten times or more. ▲

14-7. Exercise 4.—Raise the eyes upward obliquely to the right. ▲

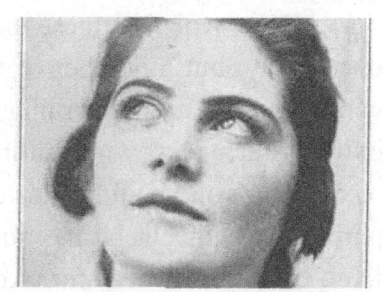

14-8. Exercise 4 (Continued).—Then stretch them obliquely downward to the left. Continue back and forth ten times or more. ▲

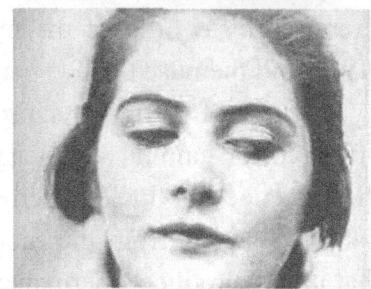

14-9. Exercise 5.—Roll the eyes around in a circle, to the left upward, to the right downward, so on around. Then reverse, rolling them the other way around. Continue until slightly tired. ▲

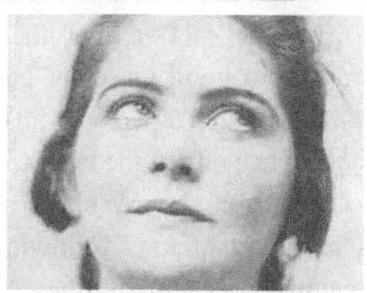

14-10. Exercise 6.—Shut the eyes tightly and vigorously, squeezing the eyelids together as firmly as possible. Open and repeat ten times or more. ▲

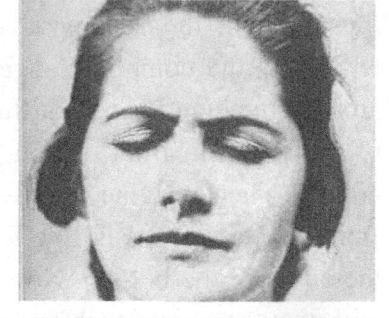

14-11. Exercise 7.—This is an exercise that should be performed without strain, and at first with only two to four repetitions at a time. Simply look cross-eyed as though trying to see the bridge of the nose with both eyes at once. ▲

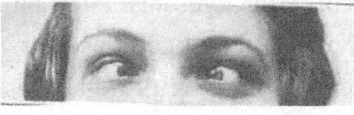

You will find these exercises very simple. Practice them not once a day, but a number of times each day. You can practice them while dressing in the morning, while undressing in the evening, while out on your walks, while sitting in the car, or even while taking your meals. But you should set aside some particular time for this special purpose, whether it be morning or evening, else they are more than likely to be crowded out. At this time you should follow the eye exercises by a little of the massage treatment described in Chapter XVII, and then use the eye bath described in Chapter XVIII.

One of the most vigorous of eye exercises, and one extremely effective for gaining voluntary control of the muscles of the eyes, is the practice of looking cross-eyed. A great many persons will naturally shrink from the thought of such an exercise from the fear that it may produce a permanent condition of strabismus.

The fact is that the ability to look cross-eyed voluntarily indicates a good muscular condition and good control of the muscles concerned, and a person with a tendency to involuntary squint will find the practice one of the best ways in the world to correct that condition.

Another very simple method of exercising the eyes will be found in a system of following lines drawn within a large circle, or an imaginary system of lines based upon any diagram, such as those illustrated in the accompanying drawings. Suppose that the circle represents the completer ange of vision attained by rolling the eyes around. Imagine, then, that this circle occupies the space on the wall of the room, in front of you, that you can see by rolling your eyes around. Then imagine a series of lines or a continuous line running from side to side, as in Eye Exercise Diagram No. 1, from the top of the circle to the bottom. Now, starting at the top, follow on the wall with your eyes just such an imaginary scheme of lines as that in the diagram. Practice this a few moments with one eye first, then with the other, finally with both eyes together, and then go on to the exercise suggested in Diagram No. 2. In Diagram No. 3 the eye starts in the center, then traces out a circular, or to be more exact, an imaginary spiral line, until the circling of the entire range of vision is attained. The head must not be moved.

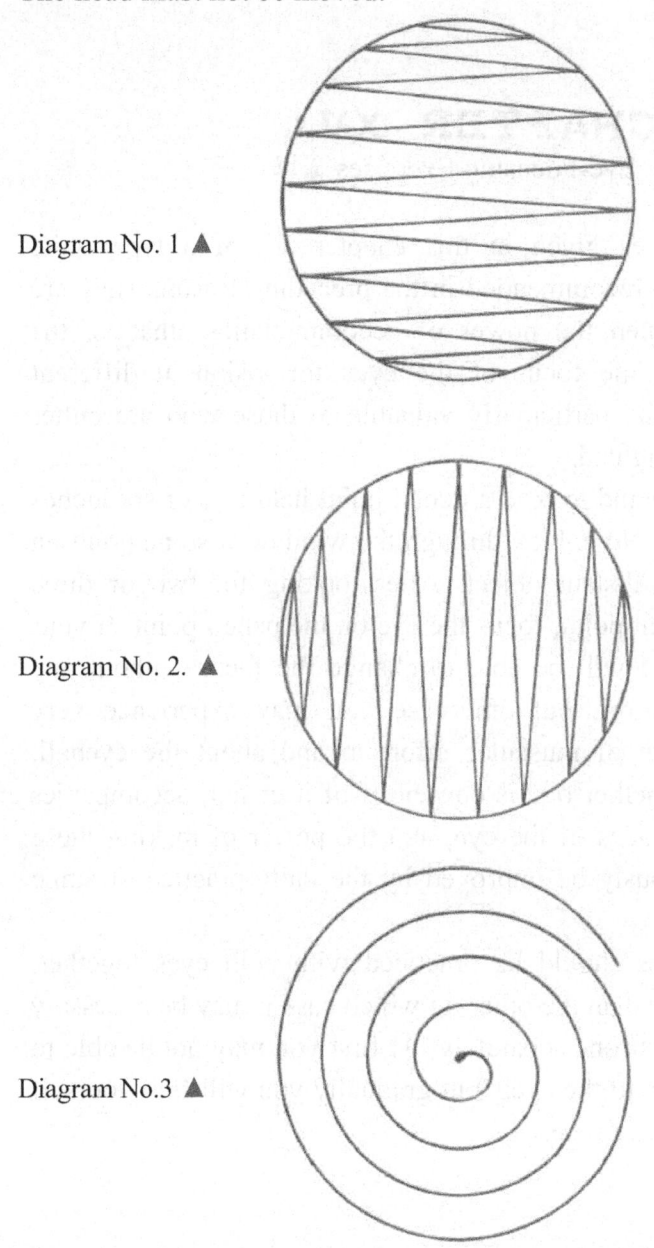

Diagram No. 1 ▲

Diagram No. 2. ▲

Diagram No.3 ▲

If you follow the eye exercises offered in the photographic illustrations there will be no need of adding these imaginary line-tracing exercises. But you may find them interesting as a change.

CHAPTER XV:
Eye-Focusing Exercises ▲

The exercises given in this chapter are of a type quite different from those recommended in the preceding lesson. They are designed to strengthen the power of accommodation, that is, the power of changing the focus of the eyes for vision at different distances, and will be particularly valuable to those who are either near-sighted or far-sighted.

Shut one eye and look at a pencil point held five or six inches in front of the other. Now, look through the window at some point on the horizon or any distant object. After looking for two or three seconds at this distant point, focus the eye on the pencil point. If your eyes are normal you will be able to change the focus without any consciousness of effort, but otherwise you may experience very clearly the sensation of muscular effort in and about the eyeball. Muscular action, whether one is conscious of it or not, accompanies all changes of the focus of the eye, and the power of making these changes must obviously be improved by the daily practice of some such exercise as this.

The exercises should be practiced with both eyes together, unless one is weaker than the other, in which case it may be necessary to practice the weaker one separately. At first you may not be able to see things very close to the eyes, but gradually you will find yourself able to diminish the distance.

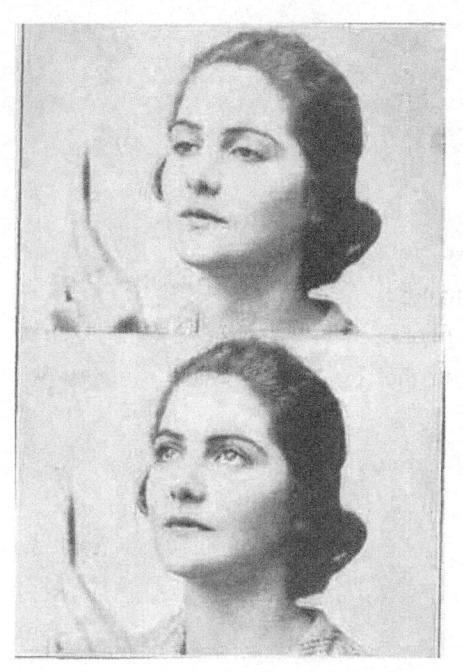

Eye Can See Clearly Now 79

15-1. An eye-focusing exercise for both eyes. (See text.) Look first at the point of a pencil held near by, as in the upper photo; then shift to a distant cloud, or some tree or building on the horizon. Immediately upon seeing the distant object, shift back again to the pencil point. ▲

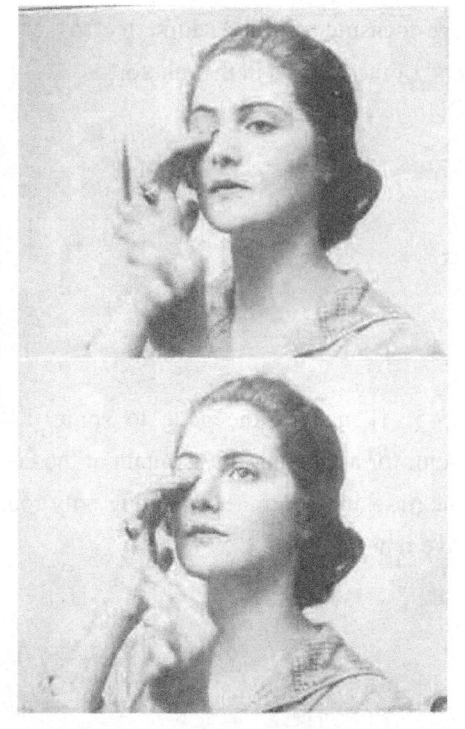

15-2. A similar eye-focusing exercise, using one eye at a time. Look at the nearby pencil point or any close object, then at some distant object; return to the pencil point and continue. ▲

15-3. Another eye-focusing exercise. Closing one eye, look at the end of the nose with the open eye, as in the upper photo, then at some distant point. Same with the other eye. ▲

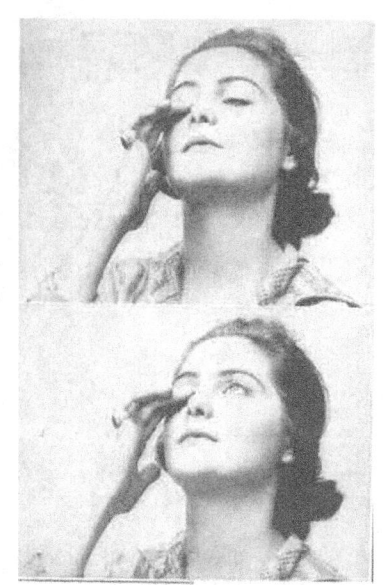

15-4. A combination eyeball exercise and eye-focusing exercise. First try to see the end of the nose as in this photo. ▲

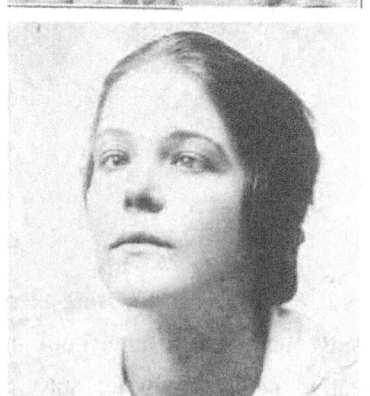

15-5. Then shift the gaze to some distant point for a moment. Look again at the end of the nose and continue, repeating only four or five times at first. ▲

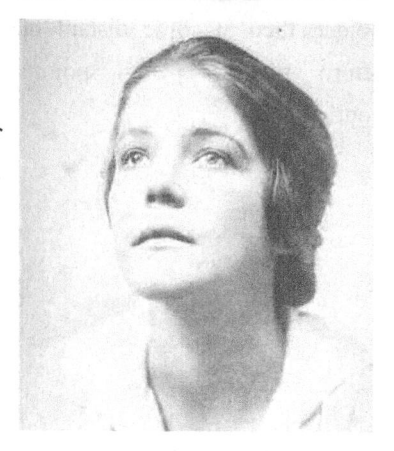

Begin by holding your pencil at whatever point you can see it most clearly, focus the eyes upon it for a moment, and then look at some distant object, such as a cloud, a tree, a house, or a chimney. You can vary the exercise, if you like, by looking at intervening distances, from a few feet up to fifty feet, one hundred feet, three hundred feet and so on. Then you can begin to hold the pencil point, thimble, needle, printed card, or whatever it is you choose to use, nearer to the eye. You will, in time, find that you can easily shift your vision from a distant object to your pencil or thimble held perhaps four or six inches in front of the eye, and see clearly and sharply at each distance.

A fairly good plan is to go to the window, and instead of using a pencil find some speck or imperfection in the glass which you can utilize as the nearby point, and then alternately shift the sight from this point to a cloud or distant tree.

Another plan is to throw the head back, shutting one eye, and with the other trying to see the end of the nose, afterward looking to the distance and then back to the end of the nose. This exercise, when practiced with both eyes together, combines the advantage of looking cross-eyed with those of rapidly changing the focus.

CHAPTER XVI:
Exercises for the Pupil of the Eye ▲

It is a comparatively simple matter to exercise the little dilator and sphincter muscles which have to do with the enlarging and diminishing of the pupil of the eye. Under normal conditions of vigor these muscles scarcely need attention. It is only when the eyes are weak, and these muscles do not respond readily in accommodating the opening to various degrees and intensities of light, that special exercise is required.

Naturally, the only practical way to exercise these muscles is to find a method of exposing the eye in rapid succession to degrees of light of varying intensity. At night this may be done by turning an electric light on and off repeatedly for a minute or two. In the daytime one can stand in a room with one window, pulling the shade down to darken the room, and then raising it and looking out of doors. In either case try to see the various objects in the room when it is darkened. It is through this attempt to see in the dark that the dilator muscles will be especially stimulated, as the pupil enlarges as much as possible to enable you to see.

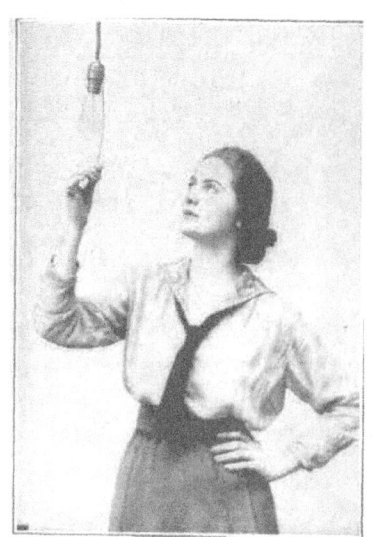

16-1. Exercising the pupil of the eye. This is best done in a dark room. At first, do not look directly at the light but at some white object, turning the light off and on at intervals of two or three seconds. You can soon accustom yourself to looking squarely at the light while turning it on and off. One minute or less will be sufficient. ▲

When the electric light is turned on, or the shade raised, the greatest stimulation will be derived from looking directly at the light, or at the sun, for an instant, provided this does not involve the sensation of eye strain or discomfort. It might not be wise, however, to do this unless you are sure that your eyes are fairly strong. You can get sufficiently good results by looking at any white object when the light is turned on, for instance, the blank page of a book. Turn the light on and off at intervals of two or three seconds. If your eyes are sensitive to artificial light it may be better to practice this exercise in the daytime, pulling down the window shade and then raising it. One or two minutes of this exercise usually should be sufficient.

CHAPTER XVII:
Eye Massage and Resistance ▲

In conjunction with the various methods for strengthening and invigorating the eyes outlined in this book, massage of the eye and adjacent tissues will be found, in many cases, to be of great practical value.

Massage is known to be beneficial in its effects upon all parts of the body. The nerves are stimulated, the blood stirred into greater and more active circulation, and the muscles and tissues generally stimulated into more vigorous life. It is now employed to advantage in many forms of disease.

The professional beauty knows these facts, and lays the greatest stress upon both facial and bodily massage, while athletic trainers rub and massage the bodies of their charges before and after any event of importance.

Why, then, should some form of modified massage not be of value in the treatment of the eyes? Of course, one can not very well massage the eyes in the same way one would a muscle, but they can certainly be strengthened and invigorated by manipulation which quickens the circulation of the blood and stimulates the nerves.

The illustration showing the "heel" of the hand over the eye shows the position for straight pressure, which is frequently very helpful in case of the acute stabbing pains that sometimes shoot through the eye as the result of straining. When there is a definite acute inflammation this treatment must not be applied, but otherwise it gives considerable relief—not only from pain but from strain and tiredness. It may be given gently in case of glaucoma, but care must be taken in this instance to observe immediate and after effects and avoid a degree of pressure that is irritating.

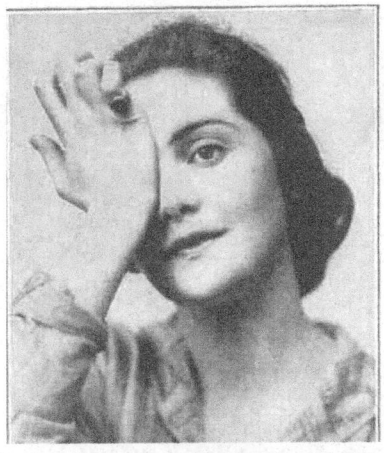

17-1. Probably the best eye massage is applied with the heel of the hand, either at the base of the thumb or opposite as in the above photo. With gentle pressure give the hand a twisting movement. At the same time, contract and relax the eyelid muscles. This is in line with the natural impulse often felt to "rub the eyes." ▲

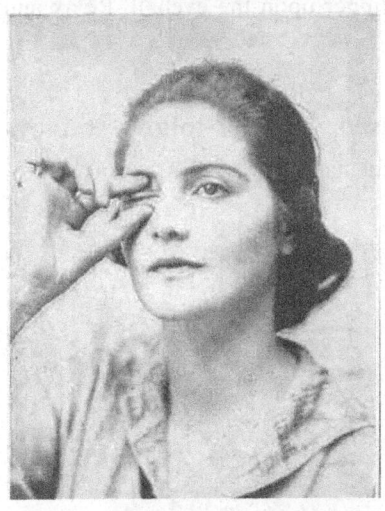

17-2. Placing the thumb and finger upon the upper and lower eyelids as illustrated, impart a very gentle massaging motion. You should gently "feel" the eyeball in applying this massage. A half a minute or less should be sufficient. ▲

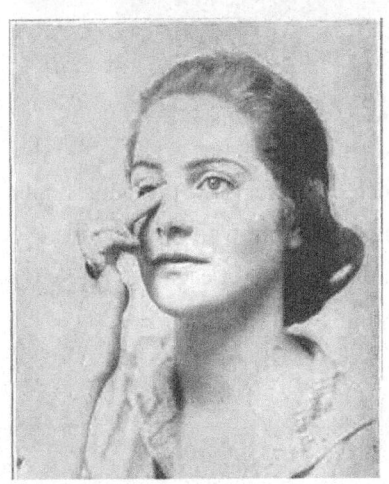

17-3. With two fingers placed one on each side of the eyeball make a gentle upward and downward movement. Use no pressure. The gentlest movement will suffice. ▲

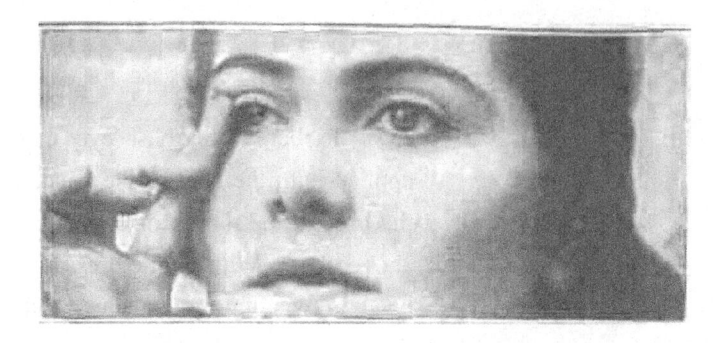

17-4. A gentle resistance exercise. Either close or partly close the right eye, placing the forefinger at the right of the eye. Then turn the eye to the right and resist very slightly with the pressure of the finger upon the eyeball. Relax and repeat a few times only. ▲

This massage treatment, if used, should follow the eye exercises. It is a good plan to follow the massage with the eye bath.

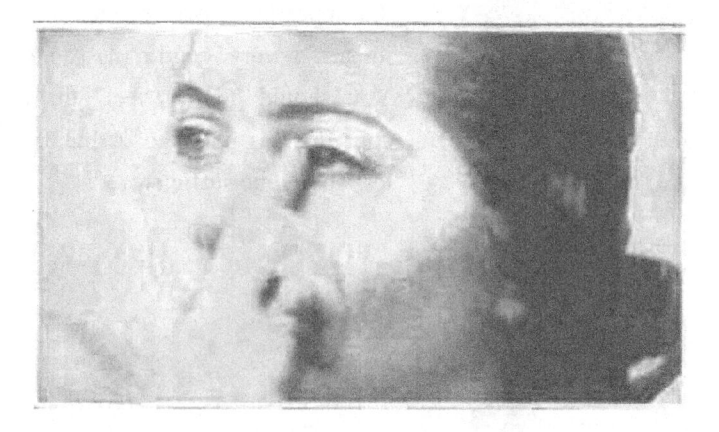

17-5. A continuation of the preceding resistance exercise. Shift the same finger to the inner side of the left eye, resisting slightly as before while turning the eye to the right. The left forefinger can be used on the left side of each eye. ▲

Other good movements are, placing the balls of the fingers between the eyeball and the bony socket above, below, and to either side, and giving gentle pressure in the opposite direction.

When the eyes are tired either hot or cold cloths may be placed over them and gentle massage given through the cloth. In this case the heel of the hand is usually better than the balls of the fingers.

When there is pain in the eye or when they are fatigued, or when there is that occasional small twitching of the eyelid, a good treatment can be given by placing the ball of one finger over the small notch felt at the edge of the eyebrow slightly inward from the center, and giving pressure here. Pressure may be given at the notch over each eye at the same time. It is usually better to give a steady pressure for at least two or three minutes. This may follow or be followed by the hot applications and gentle massage. A similar treatment may be given to the notch at the very edge of the bony socket immediately in the center below the eye.

The ball of each forefinger or of each thumb may be applied to the inner edge of the eye, but above the margin of the lower lid where the drainage canal is situated. Steady pressure may be applied here in case of eyeache or a headache resulting from eye strain.

CHAPTER XVIII:
The Eye Bath ▲

It is a good plan to follow the massage of the eyes with an "eye bath." A *weak* solution of salt and water or a dilute solution of boric acid and water, is the best for this purpose, under ordinary conditions. These solutions must on no account be *strong*. The water must not be brine, nor the boric acid solution too strong. The water should usually be cool, or lukewarm; but the temperature must depend upon circumstances. In certain inflammatory conditions of the eye, it is often advisable to have the water quite cold, while, on the other hand, in all injuries and local affection which render the eye sore or tender, it is best to bathe it in warm or hot water—at least at first. The bath, as a rule, should not last more than twenty or thirty seconds for each eye, and should be followed by a blinking of the eye—which, however, will probably follow automatically.

The eye bath may be taken in two ways. The first method is to fill an ordinary bowl with water, hold the breath, immerse the face in the water, and then open and close the eyes a number of times while the eyes are well under water. This may be repeated two or three times. This is the first method, and while it has the disadvantage of wetting the whole face, has the advantage of lack of suction, which the second method entails.

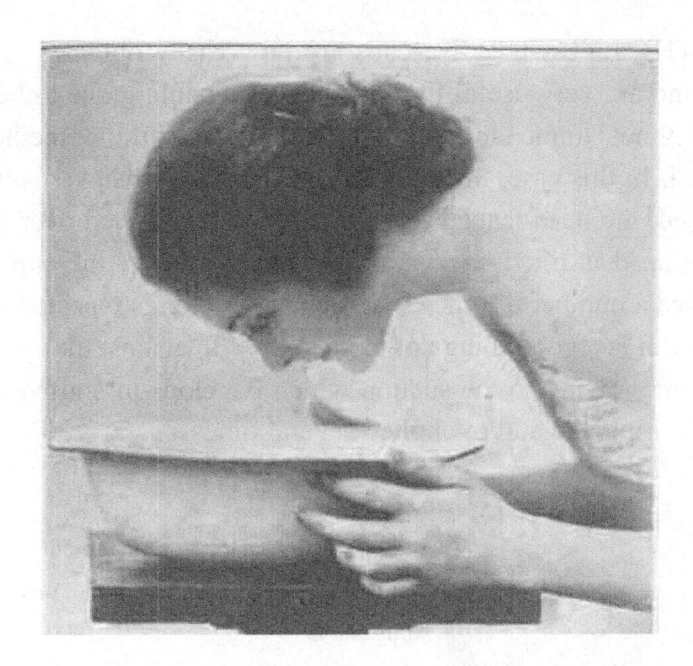

18-1. For taking the eye bath, the simplest plan is to fill an ordinary wash bowl with a weak solution of salt water or dilute boric acid. ▲

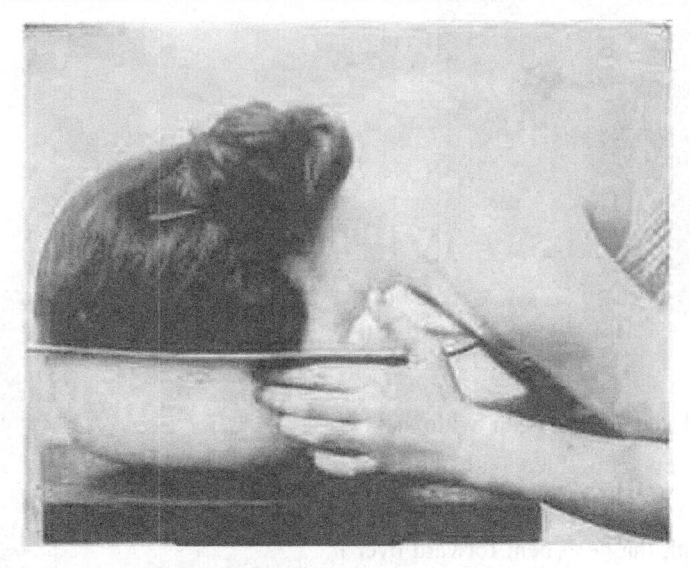

18-2. Taking the eye bath in a basin. Immerse the face in the salt water or boric acid solution and open the eyes under water, then move them from side to side, up and down, and roll them around. ▲

THE EYE-CUP. Eye-cups are now easily obtained, at a low figure, and are very useful little appliances, enabling one to bathe the eyes, without immersing the whole face, as in the method just described. In this case, the eye-cup is filled with whatever solution is to be used, the head leaned forward and the cup placed over the eye; then the head is tilted backward, and the eye under the cup opened and closed a number of times. The same operation is repeated with the other eye. It is a good thing not to keep the cup against the eye for too long a time, owing to the suction which develops in consequence. It should be removed and re-applied several times.

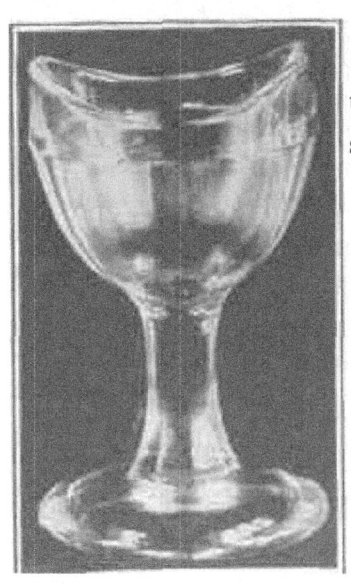

18-3. The eye-cup. A convenient device for taking the eye bath with a minimum of solution. ▲

18-4. Taking an eye bath with the eye-cup. The eye-cup filled with the desired solution is so placed as to fit the eye socket with the head bent forward over it. Then tip the head back as in the illustration and open the eye and move it about in the solution. ▲

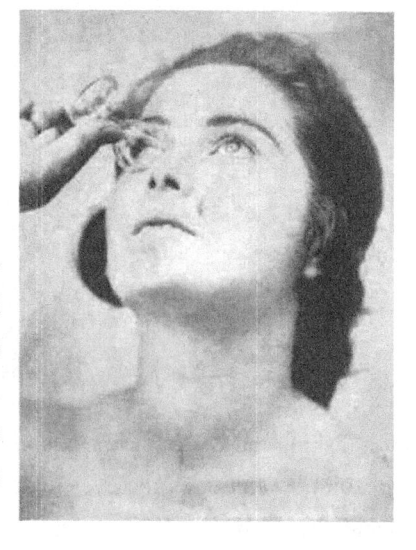

As regards medicinal substances to be used in the water, there are but few of these which can be recommended. A small percentage of salt is often strengthening to the eyes, but a heavy brine is irritating and injurious. A dilute solution of boric acid is often beneficial, as it tends to cleanse the eye and wash out irritating substances. Apart from these solutions, it is safe to say that ordinarily, the further the patient keeps from "eye lotions" and concoctions of that sort, the better. These eye baths should have the effect of strengthening and stimulating the eyes in a wholesome, hygienic manner, without irritation. Cases of weak and dull eyes are especially helped by them, and they are helpful in practically every case of eye disease and defect, where they are not distinctly contra-indicated.

CHAPTER XIX:
Eye Strength Through Sunlight ▲

Here is presented a most remarkable discovery to the effect that the rays of the sun have not only a beneficial, but a curative effect upon the eyes. The physician who conducted these researches, and who affirms the validity of these statements, does not attempt to explain this benignant influence of the sunlight, but fact is attested by numerous proofs.

The author, however, suggests caution in attempting any home treatment of this kind. The policy of "safety first" has come to be a recognized principle of modern life, and it would undoubtedly be wise to experiment carefully with radical measures of this sort. Any one can experiment with sun-gazing in the early morning or late afternoon, but caution is suggested in attempting to outstare the noonday sun in June. The burning glass should never be used by inexperienced persons.

While it is recognized in a general way that light is good for the eyes, most people entertain a fear of what they call "strong light." For this reason, as well as because the light often causes them actual discomfort, people protect their eyes from the sunlight with smoked or amber glasses and broad-brimmed hats and parasols, while persons working under artificial light use eye-shades and similar devices. All this is, to a large extent, superstition.

The eyes need no protection either from the light of the sun or from any other light. No artificial light can equal the rays of the sun in intensity, and the sunlight, far from being harmful, is the best thing in the world for the eyes. The eyes were made to react to the light, and in its absence they deteriorate and become weak. Fishes which live in sunless caves become blind; miners and people living in dark tenements develop all sort of eye troubles. Their eyes become increasingly sensitive to the light-rays until after a time they cannot look at strong light at all without pain. Then they are advised not to do so, but to rest the eyes by remaining in a dark room until they have recovered! As a matter of fact, the eyes are weak just *because* they have lacked the benefit of the sun's rays; and what they need more than anything else, in order to get well, is the thing of which they have been deprived. Sunlight is one of the best curative agents we can employ for the eye. Persons with weak and defective eyes should look in the direction of the sun every day, until they are able to look straight at it without pain or injury.

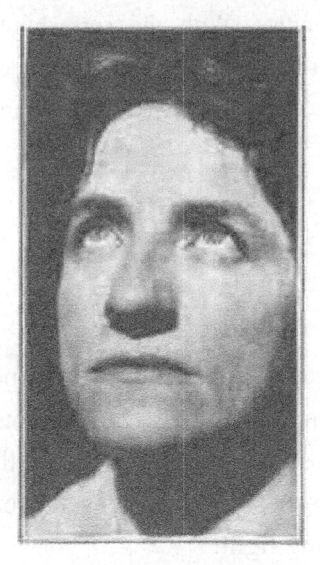

19-1. Persons with normal sight can look directly at the sun without injury or discomfort. Note that the eyes are wide open, with no evidence of pain and no watering. ▲

Not only is it beneficial to look at the sun, but in most diseases of the eyes the sun's rays concentrated upon them by means of a burning glass exert a remarkably curative effect. The following are examples of hundreds of similar cases that might be cited:

A man suffering from inflammation of the eyelids was unable to attend to his work, because, as soon as he left the house and went into the sunlight the discomfort he experienced was so great that he could not keep his eyes open, and had to return home. He had been in this condition for more than fifteen years, and had received all kinds of treatment from many physicians. After a few treatments with the burning glass he was able to return to his work without further trouble. Another man suffering from trachoma was unable to open his eyes in the sunlight and therefore had great difficulty in finding his way about. One treatment enabled him to open his eyes and go into the sunlight without discomfort.

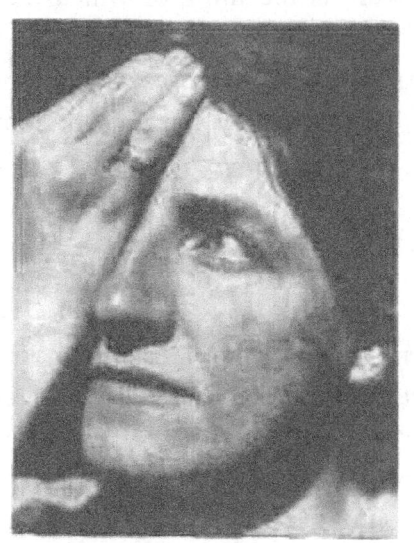

19-2. Demonstrating again that the normal eye can regard the orb of day without injury. With the sun shining almost directly into her eye, the subject reads the Snellen test card with normal vision. ▲

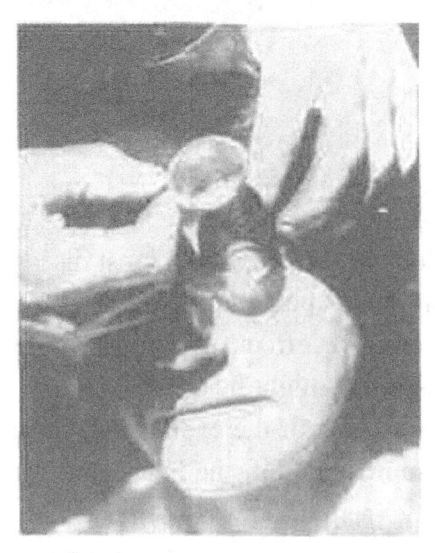

These cases are interesting, not only in themselves, but because they strikingly illustrate the baselessness of the present fear of strong light.

19-3. Concentrating the rays of the sun upon the eyeball with a lens or "burning glass," demonstrated to be an effective curative measure in conjunctivitis, iritis, ulcers of the cornea and other diseases of the eyes. ▲

CHAPTER XX:
Constitutional Improvement for Strengthening the Eyes ▲

If your eyes are weak or your sight impaired in any manner whatsoever, one of the first requirements for improvement is to build up a better state of the general health.

It may have been your experience, just as it has been that of countless others, that signs of weakness of the eyes, failing of the sight, twitching of the eyelids and a smarting and burning sensation have accompanied a condition of depleted vitality. After your health has been restored you have found that your eyes grew stronger and better, giving you little or no further trouble.

Practically every one has had some such experiences. At all events, it is undeniably true that the condition of the general health is very largely reflected in the eyes, just as it is in the voice, in the complexion, in one's whole mental and physical bearing. As soon as you build vitality, strengthen the nervous system and improve the condition of the blood, the eyes acquire new vigor.

The reason for all this is obvious. The eyes depend upon the blood supply. If it is of the proper quantity and purity it will tend to keep these organs vigorous, just as all parts of the body are thus kept vigorous. If the blood is in poor condition, filled with impurities and sluggishly circulated, then you can not expect to keep your eyes, or any other part of your body, in the best condition. It is for this reason that good digestion, active elimination and general functional vigor must be considered if you wish to improve the condition of your eyes. In other words, constitutional treatment is necessary.

One of the first lessons for every man, woman and child to learn is that illness is one's own fault. It is purely a matter of cause and effect. Sickness comes as an inevitable result of habits and conditions of life which would logically produce such a result. Health is merely the effect of normal and natural habits of life. If you live in accordance with the laws of Nature you make illness practically impossible.

The truth is that it requires more energy to be sick than to be well. In a state of health the organs function properly, naturally and easily. There is no special effort upon the part of any one of them. Life proceeds smoothly and easily. But when one is sick the body has to struggle against poisons, against various handicaps, and the work of each organ of the body becomes a serious effort. Sickness means hard work for the body. Good health means freedom from all these troubles. It is, therefore, far easier to be well than to be sick.

If you have strength enough to resist illness and still live, you certainly will have energy enough to recover normal health, and to keep it. But you cannot secure health in a drug store. You cannot build health simply by conversing with a physician and paying him regrettable sums of money. You can build health only by obeying the laws of Nature, by cultivating habits and conditions such as will increase your strength, help your organs to function more perfectly and smoothly, and purify and improve the condition of your blood.

The cornerstones of health may be said to be exercise, air, food and sleep.

Exercise is probably the most neglected of all these vital health essentials. The first characteristic of all life is movement or the capacity for movement. You see an insect, a reptile, a lobster or any other animal lying motionless, and you wonder whether it is alive or dead. Perhaps you poke it with a stick. If it moves you know that it is alive. Our lives are based upon the capacity for movement. This applies not merely to the muscles which move the body about, but to the muscular organs which maintain the vital processes, such as the heart, stomach and blood-vessels, which have muscles in their walls to keep the contents circulating.

Forty per cent or more—that is to say, from two-fifths to one-half—of the weight and bulk of the body in a state of health and vigor is made up of muscular tissue. Most of the food is consumed in the muscles. It is inevitable, therefore, that a healthy state of the muscular system is a prime condition of what we call health. We are essentially muscular creatures. Therefore, to permit our muscles to degenerate and deteriorate means not only a loss of strength, but it means a poor and weak circulation, a loss of tone in all the organs, and consequently a general impairment of the health.

You will see from all this that muscular activity is absolutely essential to health. Inactivity means stagnation. Stagnation not merely of the muscles, but of the blood and of all those vital forces which together make up what we call life. Out-of-door exercise is undoubtedly the best. You should make it a point to get enough of it. But whether you can spend much time outdoors or not, you should certainly take enough exercise of a strength-building character in your own home, or in your own room, to maintain the muscular system in a state of full development and normal vigor. More detailed consideration of the subject of exercise for constitutional purposes will be given in the next chapter.

CHAPTER XXI:
Exercises for Constitutional Improvement ▲

The value and necessity of exercise as a factor in constitutional improvement has already been pointed out. Every one needs a proper amount of exercise for the sake of the general health, irrespective of the effect upon his eyes.

Without going too deeply into the physiology of exercise, it may be said that there are two general results to be gained from any good system of physical training. In other words, exercise may affect one in two ways. It may have chiefly a muscle-building value. Or it may have what is commonly called a constitutional or health-building value. Muscle-building exercises are intended chiefly to build strength and enlarge the muscles. Constitutional exercises chiefly affect the heart, the lungs, the vital organs generally, and, in consequence, the purity and quality of the blood.

Now, nearly all exercises partake of this twofold purpose. They strengthen and enlarge the muscles and, at the same time, they build up the general health through their effect upon the heart and lungs, the digestive and eliminative systems. That is why almost any form of activity, if one secures enough of it, is likely to fulfill all requirements in both these respects. At the same time there are some exercises which are particularly of the muscle-building type and are only slightly constitutional in their influence. There are others which have only a small muscle-building value, being useful mainly because of their effect in toning up the vital organs.

Editor's Note: The following pages in the paperback and pdf have been formatted for convenient photocopying and posting in your home or office. Electronic book readers may download them at www.agelessadept.com/resources

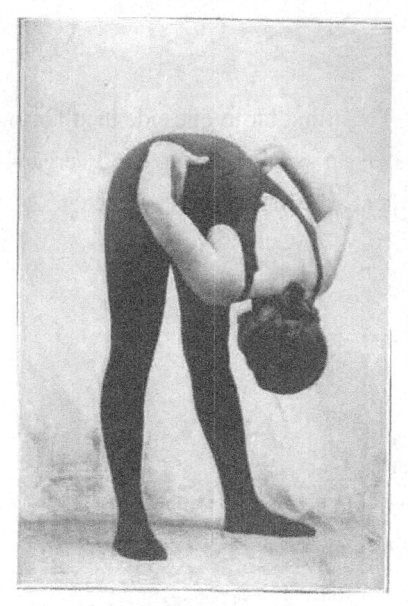

←Exercise 1.—With the hands at the hips bend far forward in the manner illustrated. Repeat five or ten times according to strength. It is best to commence with a few repetitions and increase the number with the increase of strength. ▲

Exercise 2.—Bend well backward in the manner illustrated. It is usually most convenient to combine exercises 1 and 2 in one movement. Repeat as desired. ▲

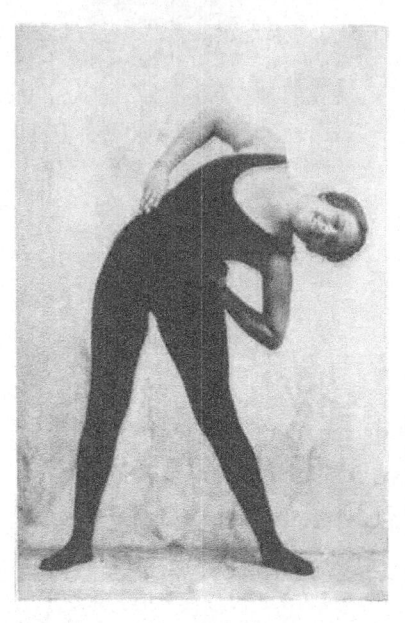

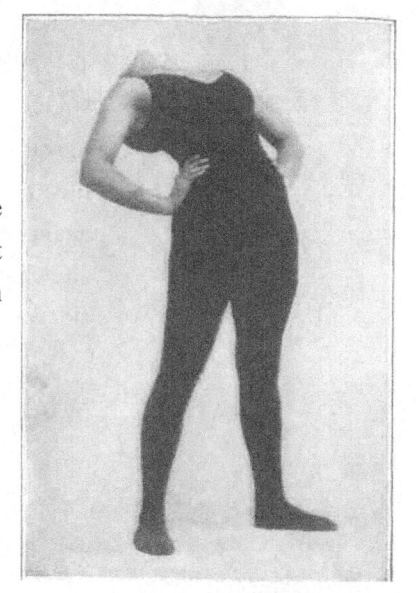

←Exercise 3.—With feet well apart to give a better base of support, bend the body far sideways, to both sides, five or ten times. ▲

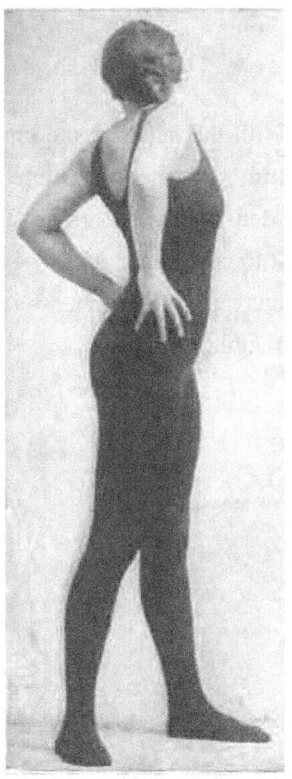

←Exercise 4.—Twist first far to one side then far to the other. This is a spine-twisting and organ-stretching movement. The more action, the better. ▲

Exercise 5→ —Fingers extended, stretch vigorously upward, lower arms, then stretch upward again. Vary by stretching forward and sideways. ▲

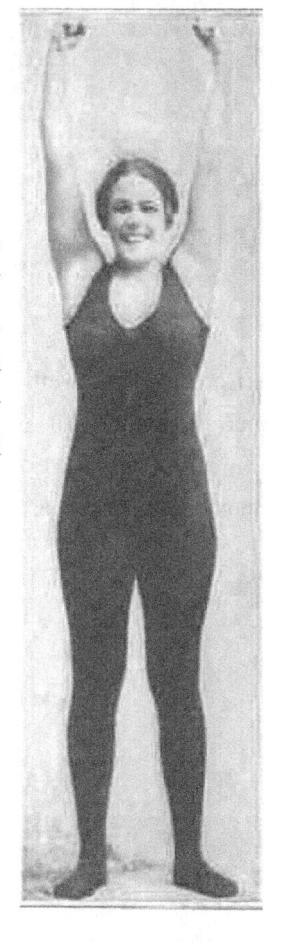

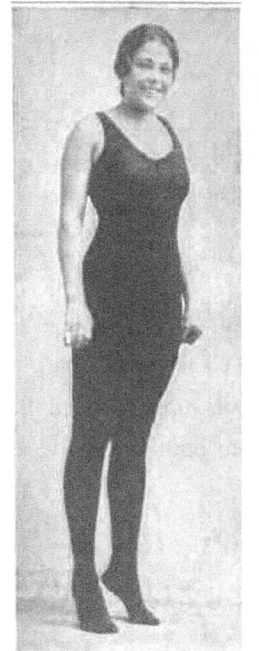

←Exercise 6.—Raise the body high on the toes as illustrated. If too easy, do it on one foot at a time. ▲

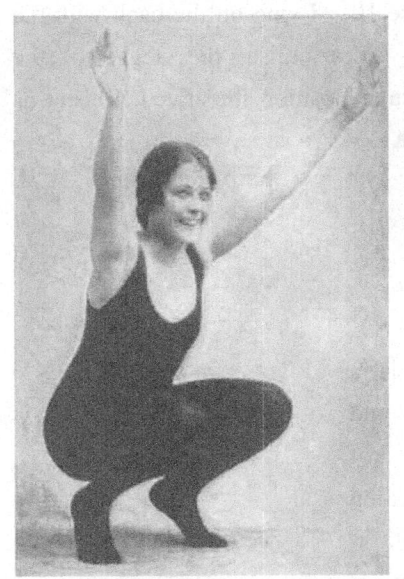

←Exercise 7.—Starting in a standing position with the arms at the sides, bend the knees and lower the body to the squatting position. It is easier to maintain balance and requires less effort if the arms are swung forward and upward as the body is being lowered, as illustrated. ▲

Exercise 8.—Bring one knee at a time upward as high as possible with a snappy, kicking movement. A little more action is secured by swinging the arms upward at the same time. Repeat five or ten times or more with each leg.→▲

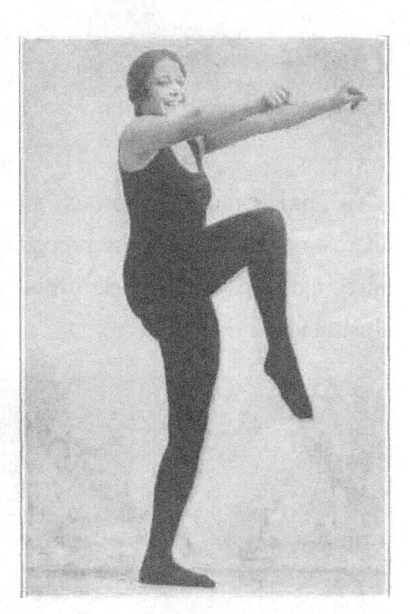

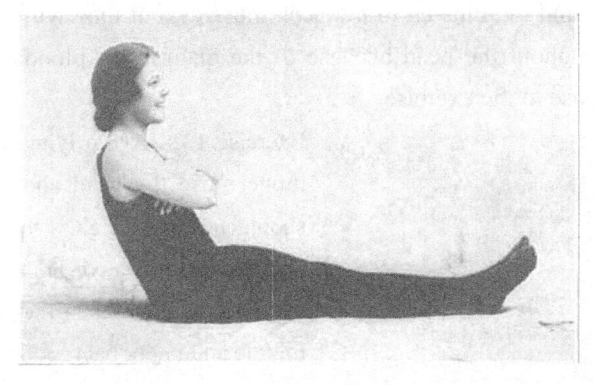

←Exercise 9.—Lying on the back with arms folded, raise body to a sitting position. Repeat according to strength and fatigue. If necessary, use a weight over the feet. ▲

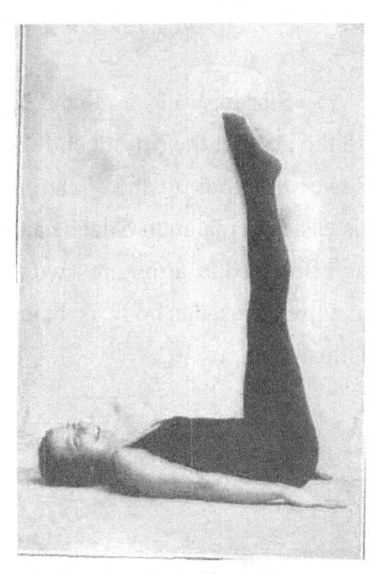

←Exercise 10.—Lying on the back with the arms at sides, raise the legs to the perpendicular position illustrated. Repeat as desired. ▲

Exercise 11. — This is a variation and extension of the preceding movement. It is a little more vigorous hut also more interesting. Continuing the preceding movement, raise the hips and back from the floor as illustrated. ▲ →

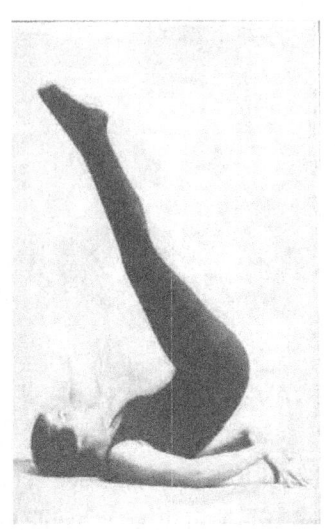

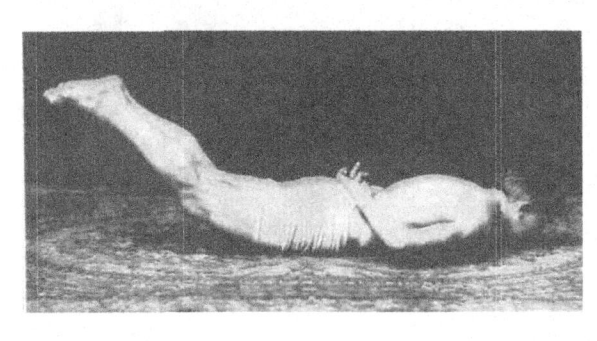

Exercise 12 —Lying prone with hands behind the back, raise feet and, if possible, the entire length of both legs as high as possible. This involves the muscles of the lower region of the back and the hips up to the neck muscles, but they will improve the circulation throughout the head because of the quantity of blood sent in this direction in response to the exercise. ▲

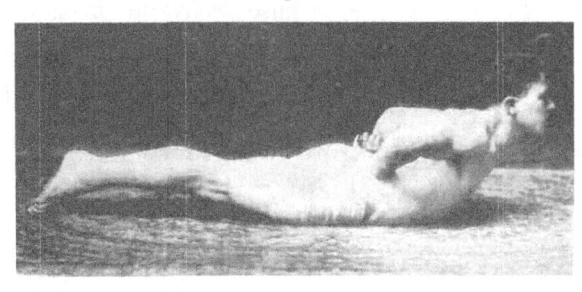

Exercise 13.—Again lying prone, raise the head and shoulders as high as possible as illustrated. This involves the muscles of the middle and upper back. ▲

Eye Can See Clearly Now 103

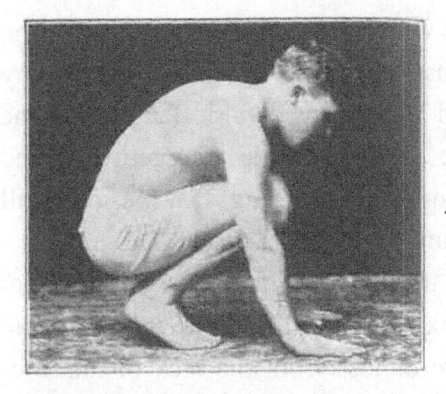

Exercise 14.—Starting from a standing position, bend down and place the hands on the floor in the manner illustrated. Then with a jumping movement, kick the feet back until the body is straight with the weight on hands and feet. (See next photo.) ▲

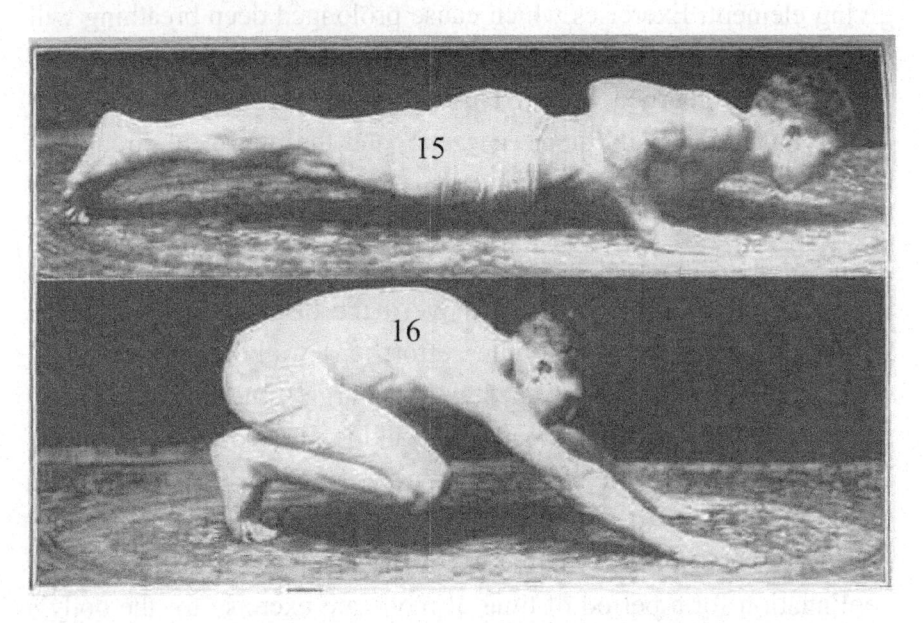

Exercises 15 and 16.—Next lower the body as shown in the upper photo. Push up and repeat until slightly tired. A variation is shown in lower photo. Keep arms stiff, straighten the legs, projecting the body forward with head well in front of supporting position of hands. Swing back, repeat. ▲

All those types of exercise which call for endurance are of the greatest value from a constitutional standpoint. In other words, any exercise which may be continued for a considerable length of time and which, therefore, keeps the heart working energetically and causes one to breathe deeply and freely during that period, will inevitably tone up the internal organs.

The shallow breathing of the inactive man or woman is not calculated to fill the blood with oxygen, and the brain and all of the structures of the body suffer more or less from the lack of this life-giving element. Exercises which cause prolonged deep breathing will naturally increase the oxygen intake until your entire body from top to toe is literally charged with it. This will make you more alive. It will make you brighter and more energetic, and the improved circulation will tend to tone up every cell and every structure of the body.

It is for this reason that a long walk is one of the best of all forms of constitutional exercise. Every time you step you lift the weight of your entire body and move it the distance of your stride. Although there may be little effort in walking, nevertheless considerable energy is consumed, and the largest muscles of the body are brought into play. It is because walking is accomplished by the largest muscles that the effort seems easy. Nevertheless it calls for a large supply of blood and of oxygen. This means increased circulation and deeper breathing. Walking for a distance, therefore, means the continuation for a period of time of moderate exercise for the body's largest muscles, without involving any strain. There is the very least expenditure of nerve-force in proportion to the physiological benefit.

There are other forms of constitutional exercise which do not involve any severe strain upon the muscles, and which are beneficial largely because of their endurance-building quality. Cycling at moderate speed, hill climbing, rowing for pleasure, horseback riding, golf, gardening, and other varieties of exercise, may be included in this class. Of course, some of these, like gardening or rowing, may be made very strenuous indeed if one wishes to exert oneself.

The exercises which we are illustrating herewith are useful both for their constitutional and their muscle-building value. They are particularly designed to keep the trunk of the body firm, strong and vigorous. Exercises that bend and twist the trunk of the body not only build up and strengthen the external muscles, thus supplying the lower trunk with strong, firm muscular walls, which prevent any prolapses or sagging of the internal organs, but they indirectly affect the internal organs, toning them up and making them far more vigorous. They also help to keep the spine and its cartilages strong, flexible and youthful.

Either the system of exercise presented herewith, or any other system which answers the same purpose, should be practiced at least once each day. It will be best to take the movements in your bedroom before dressing. If taken in the morning, they will wake you up and warm you up, so that a cold bath will be not an ordeal but a pleasure. You will find it advantageous to give the skin of the entire body a brisk rubbing following the exercises and preceding your bath. If you do not find it convenient to take the exercises in the morning, however, they may be taken either late in the afternoon or in the evening—a half hour before retiring.

Special attention is called to the exercises for the neck which are illustrated. There are two ways in which they are especially valuable: first, in improving the circulation about the neck and head; and second, in improving the upper spine, or, to be more exact, the cervical spine.

The question of active circulation is always important. These neck exercises will not only affect the neck itself, strengthening and building up the neck muscles, but they will improve the circulation throughout the head because of the quantity of blood sent in this direction in response to the exercise.

Congestion about the neck is known to produce a "fullness" in the head with consequent congestion in and about the eyes. Measures which relieve this condition will naturally tend to lessen the strain upon the eyes themselves, making for more perfect and easier sight.

Deep breathing, water drinking and relaxation, as well as exercise, are useful for this purpose. Conscious relaxation of the neck muscles with deep breathing will often relieve congestion in the head very quickly, but active exercise promoting a vigorous circulation is one of the most effective means known for overcoming either a state of congestion or an anemic condition of any part of the body.

These neck exercises will also tend to keep the upper spine flexible and in normal alignment. Exercise for spinal strength and flexibility is, perhaps, even more important, generally speaking, than exercise for muscular development, for the reason that the spine would otherwise tend to become rigid, and the little cartilages or cushion-like disks between the vertebræ hardened and compressed. Exercise will prevent this, keeping these cushions elastic and healthy. Furthermore, any displacement of the vertebræ causes a pinching of the spinal cord, or spinal nerves, and consequent interference with the currents of nerve force, with more or less derangement of various functions of the body. Osteopaths claim to accomplish very marked results in many cases of eye trouble through the proper mechanical adjustment of the spine and the freeing of the nervous impulses. Proper neck exercise will prevent adhesions of the vertebræ and tend to keep the upper spine in such perfect alignment that the spinal cord is free from any disturbing factors of this kind.

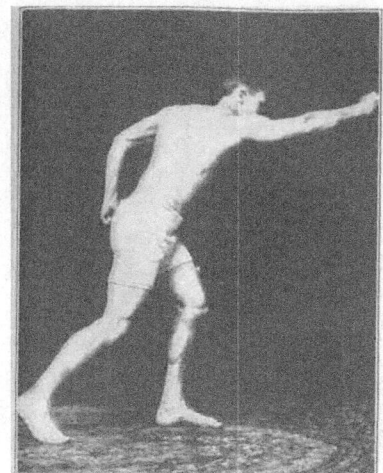

Exercise 17.—A vigorous and stimulating exercise is found in shadow boxing as shown in the above photo. Strike out forward vigorously first with one fist and then with the other, continuing to alternate until slightly tired. ▲

Exercise 18.—The "stationary run." A running action without going forward. A splendid constitutional exercise, inducing free respiration and perspiration. Excellent for finishing up any type of indoor exercise. ▲

Exercise 19.—A neck resistance exercise. Placing one hand back of the head, bring the head backward, resisting the movement with the hand in the manner illustrated. Five to ten movements.

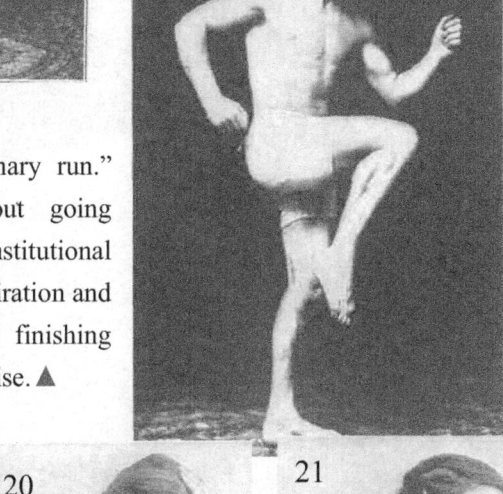

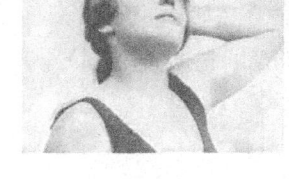

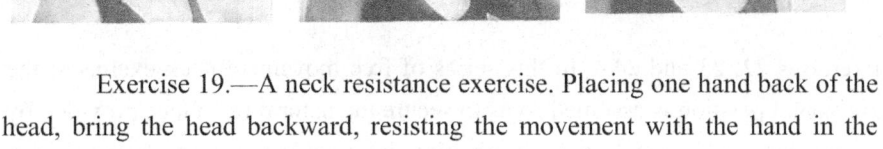

Exercise 20.—Neck exercise. Place hand against forehead and bring head forward and downward against resistance.

Exercise 21.—A simple neck exercise. Bring the head first far to one side, then to the other, placing it upon the shoulder on each side. Vary by a head-circling movement, and neck-twisting movement. ▲

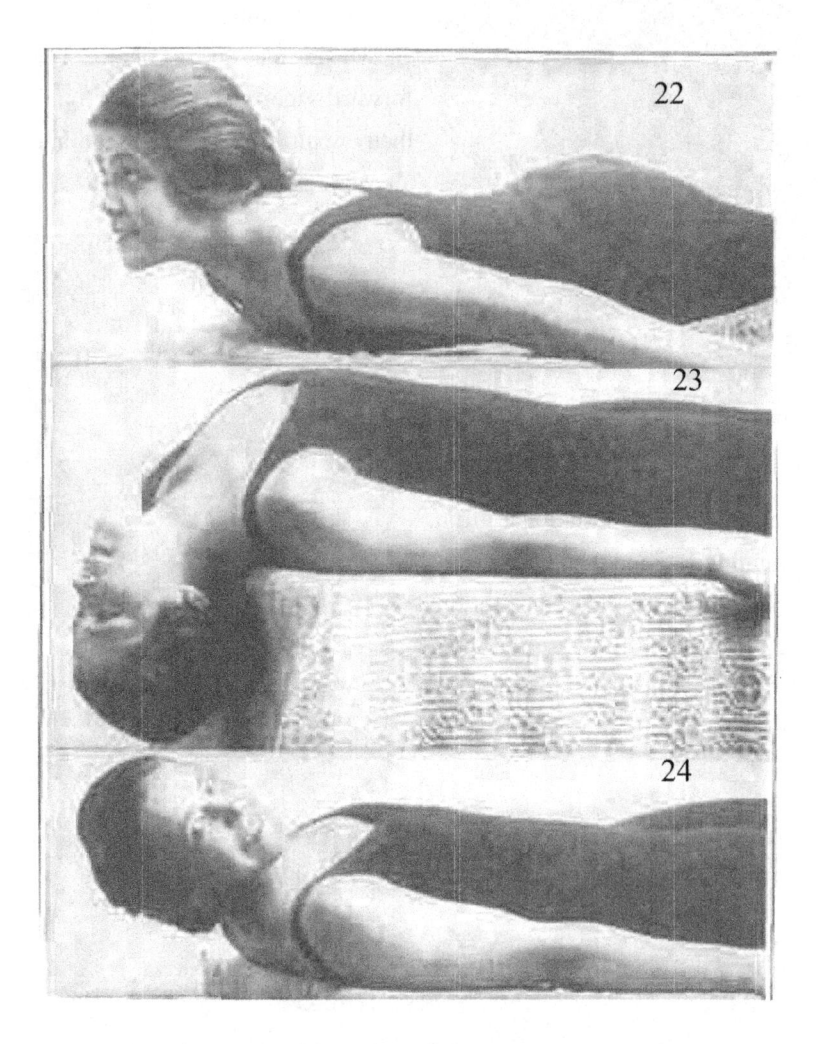

Exercises 22, 23 and 24.—In this series of free movement neck exercises, the horizontal position is assumed so as to secure the natural resistance provided by the weight of the head. In the first position, lying upon the stomach, the head is first lowered as far as possible and then raised high, as in the upper photo. In the next exercise, lying on the back, the head is first lowered as shown, and then raised straight upward and brought over the chest. In the last exercise (lower photo), the raising of the head is combined with a head-turning or neck-twisting action, very valuable for its effect upon the vertebrae of the upper spine. ▲

If you have not been accustomed to muscular exercise, a word of caution is necessary in order that you may not overdo the work the first day, and thereby produce a condition of lameness and stiffness of the muscles that is likely to be very discouraging. Enthusiasm in the beginning may lead one to take too much exercise. It is best to try only about half as much as you think you could comfortably do to start with. Never carry any exercise to the point of pronounced fatigue. As you get stronger you can increase the vigor of your movements.

If you should experience any lameness or stiffness of the muscles, the local application of hot water, or a complete hot bath, will give relief, especially if followed by energetic rubbing of the parts. In any case, the soreness will disappear in a few days and should not prevent your continuing with the exercise.

It is, of course, understood that all exercises will be taken with the windows open, so that you may have the advantage of fresh, pure air. Much of the benefit of your exercise will be lost if you breathe stale or stagnant air while you are taking it. Much of the benefit and energy that you derive from your exercises will also depend upon how much energy you put into them. Exercise vigorously. Put life, vim, determination into every movement. Ten or fifteen minutes energetically spent in these exercises will keep you vigorous and fit.

In addition, try to spend at least two or three hours a day in the open air. It may be well to start with a walk of one or two miles. Then increase the distance by a quarter of a mile each day until you are covering anywhere from five to six miles and upward. If in addition to the vigor-building exercises which are illustrated you will make it a point to take at least one good walk each day, you will have established for yourself an ideal scheme of physical culture.

Editor's Note: In practicing these exercises, some readers may notice similarities to the Five Tibetan Rejuvenation Rites, a system of exercises reported to be more than 2,500 years old which were first publicized by Peter Kelder in a 1939 publication titled *The Eye of Revelation*.

CHAPTER XXII:
Eating for Health and Strength ▲

If your eyes depend largely upon the condition of your general health and your general health depends very largely upon the condition of your stomach, you will see that it is highly important that you make no serious errors in the matter of what, when and how you eat.

What you eat is important. Your sustenance and strength depend upon it. But there are other important factors in the food problem. The question of how you eat, how much you eat and how often you eat requires nearly as much consideration, and people go wrong in these matters, perhaps, even more often than in regard to what they eat.

The first thing to learn is to follow your appetite. This means not only that you should eat when you are hungry, but also that you should not eat when you are not hungry. The greatest dietetic crime in the world is eating without appetite. Do not eat merely because the custom of the country calls for three meals per day at stated hours. If you are not hungry when meal time comes, or if you are excited, nervous, sick, or for any other reason without an appetite, then do not think of eating. Wait until appetite appears.

In other words, you should put your stomach on a natural and not on a forced regime. To force food down your throat when you do not desire it and cannot enjoy it means that you are placing an unnatural burden upon your stomach. If you are not hungry and your stomach seems a little bit upset, then drink water. The quickest relief for any form of stomach trouble is found in the drinking of hot water. This is an old-fashioned, old woman's remedy, but the best in the world. If you are "sick at your stomach" and the hot water induces vomiting, this will be the best thing that could possibly happen, for it will relieve you of the burden of the fermenting and poisonous load. And if the drinking of more water is followed by further vomiting, it will mean that the stomach has been well washed out. You will then quickly recover.

In any case the drinking of hot water has a tendency to flush or wash out the stomach, as well as the entire alimentary canal, particularly if you drink enough of it. Nothing in the world is so effective in the case of indigestion or loss of appetite, as several cups of hot water, taken at intervals of five or ten minutes, or even more frequently, if you can take it faster. I mention this for the sake of any emergency in which you may have lost your appetite or suffered from temporary indigestion. You will find that hot water, taken before meals, will improve your power of assimilation. It is to be hoped, however, that you will not need even this simple treatment for this purpose. If you have no appetite, the omission of one or two meals can be depended upon to give you an appetite such as even a child might have reason to envy.

Do not think that you must eat three times a day irrespective of appetite just because farmers and piano-movers have that kind of an appetite. For many people, especially office workers, the two-meal-per-day plan is far superior. You may take your meals either morning and evening, or noon and evening, as you choose. This is no untried theory. Millions of people eat such a light breakfast that it is practically no breakfast at all—merely coffee and rolls. In fact such a meal is *worse* than none at all. Thousands of others have found by experiment that the two-meal-per-day plan means a better appetite, better assimilation and consequently better health.

Almost as bad as eating without an appetite is eating too fast. Do not swallow your food without thorough chewing. The work of digestion is commenced in the mouth, through the treatment of the food with saliva. You should try to chew your food to a liquid before passing it on to the stomach.

On the subject of what you eat one may well hesitate to give any sweeping advice. There is no special menu or diet that will suit every one. It is not strictly true that "what is one man's meat is another man's poison," and yet there is a small measure of truth in this old saying. Do not eat anything advised by dietetic experts as ideal if you cannot enjoy it. On the other hand, do not follow the course of eating "palate ticklers" to the exclusion of plain and substantial foods.

If you have a normal and natural appetite this should dictate as to your food requirements. To a large extent the entire problem of diet may be narrowed down to the question of eating natural foods, as against those which are too much refined, or tampered with, in the process of preparation.

For instance, take the case of wheat. Wheat is a perfect food just as it is grown. It will nourish every part of the body. In the making of white flour, however, much of the best nutrition in the wheat is thrown away to be fed to stock.

A similar food crime is committed in the polishing of rice. The best part of the rice is in the natural light brown coating. When this is removed in the polishing process, leaving practically pure starch, rice is no longer an adequate or satisfactory food. The same thing applies to the refining of sugar. White granulated, or fine white powdered sugar, does not contain the nourishing elements found in the juice of the sugar cane from which it has been made.

To a large extent, the nutrition loss involved in the refinement of food is due to the wastage of the mineral salts. Old books on dietetics, after discussing the importance of protein, fats and carbohydrates (sugar and starch), were accustomed to refer to these mineral salts under the collective term of "ash," and then to dismiss them. These organic minerals form only a very small percentage of any food, but they are a vitally important percentage, nevertheless. Because they are limited in quantity it is all the more important that they should not be eliminated from any of our foods.

Not only are mineral salts lost in the commercial manipulation of flour, rice, sugar, corn and other foods, but they are often lost, also, in the kitchen. The woman who boils her potatoes, cauliflower, peas, beans and other vegetables and then throws the water down the drain commits an equally serious food crime, inasmuch as these mineral salts are, to a large extent, dissolved in the water and thus lost when the latter is thrown away. What to do about it? These vegetables should be cooked in no more water than is necessary, and simmered down so that only a moderate amount of juice, which should be served and eaten with them, is left. Don't follow the cookbooks that tell you to boil your vegetables and then "drain." Too much cannot be said about the criminal stupidity of this wastage of iron, lime, phosphorus and the many other organic mineral salts which Nature has so carefully built into the structure of plant life. The same consideration applies to draining water from other foods.

To make this discussion of food as brief as possible, therefore, it is earnestly recommended that you endeavor to follow the plan of eating foods in their natural condition as nearly as possible. If cooked, they should be as unchanged as possible. Honey is a more perfect, more digestible and more satisfactory form of sweetening than sugar. Brown sugar, being less refined, is better than white sugar.

As foods contain elements which are destroyed by cooking, the diet should contain a liberal proportion of raw foods, such as lettuce, celery, watercress, onions, peppers, tomatoes and fruits. Fruits not only help digestion, but they are especially valuable for supplying mineral salts.

The question of meat eating is one which may be left to the individual with the caution that the use of large quantities of meat is neither desirable nor necessary to health. Nearly every one would do better to eat one-fourth of the amount of meat which he consumes. It may even be just as well to eliminate meat entirely, if one uses a sufficiency of eggs, cheese, milk or buttermilk in the diet. Lentils, beans and peas are also valuable protein foods, and may be used as substitutes for meat.

Milk is the ideal food for infants and young children. It should continue to form the most important part of the diet of young children up to six or eight years of age, one quart a day being required for each child. Eggs are a substantial protein food and for tissue building may be classed with meat, fish, poultry, cheese, milk and buttermilk. Many men and women who do not care for milk will find buttermilk, or fermented milk, which answers the same nutrition requirements, more palatable and agreeable.

Constipation is an almost universal problem. It is invariably the direct result of improper diet and irrational habits of life. Given proper muscular activity, a natural diet and a sufficiency of water, constipation would be a rare condition.

What then is the victim of this stubborn and chronic complaint to do about it? The first thing is to revise the diet, using natural foods and especially a considerable amount of fruit and raw green salads. White bread is probably the greatest enemy of the constipation victim. An immediate change to whole-wheat, or graham, flour and such whole-grain cereals as oatmeal and shredded wheat will be helpful. Rice, tapioca and spaghetti are likewise constipating. Macaroni, or spaghetti, with cheese, is particularly so, but when spaghetti and macaroni are served in the Italian style, with a plentiful sauce made of olive oil, tomatoes and onions, this objection is practically eliminated.

The drinking of a sufficient amount of water is an important factor in preventing constipation. The hot water suggested earlier in the chapter is very effective indeed. Laxatives or cathartics should never be used because of the detrimental after effects. They tend to make the condition more stubborn. An enema should be used when necessary, although even an enema should be regarded as an emergency treatment. The refined mineral oil, which is sometimes known as Russian oil, and sometimes as liquid petrolatum, offers a very satisfactory means of relief and prevention. It is not assimilated, and serves merely as a lubricant.

The condition of the alimentary canal is such an important factor in the preservation of health that the above suggestions should he very carefully studied and assiduously followed. Keep at peace with your stomach and avoid constipation, and you will have little or no trouble in building up that condition of vigorous health which is conducive to the strength of your eyes.

Editor's Note: For more information on a transition diet, plus food to keep you ageless and fit to breed, check out *The Man Who Lived Forever*, and *A Clean Cell Never Dies*

CHAPTER XXIII:
Eye Rest Through Sleep ▲

The health-building, strength-restoring influence of sleep is an important factor in those cases in which the condition of the eyes is particularly concerned.

Sleep restores the reserves of nerve force and gives an opportunity for exhausted tissues to rebuild and refresh themselves, and at the same time usually affords rest for the eyes. This is not always true, however, because one can strain the eyes during sleep. Persons with eye trouble, as well as all others who do not get the proper amount of rest from their sleep, should palm before retiring, in the manner described in "Errors of Refraction: Their Cure." How long the relaxation thus induced will continue in the individual case it is impossible to say, but some persons report great benefit from this practice.

Opinions vary as to the amount of sleep required. The truth is that different individuals vary in this respect. It is a well-understood principle among students of the subject that duration of sleep is not as important for constitutional purposes as depth of sleep. In other words, many hours of light sleep are not as refreshing as half that number of hours of profound slumber. Great depth of sleep means complete mental relaxation, whereas light sleep may mean dreams, or a degree of mental activity bordering on dreamland, which does not yield the same complete relaxation and the same degree of recuperation.

There are two primary factors involved in healthful sleep. First, the surrounding conditions, and second, the condition of the slumberer himself.

Darkness and quiet are essential to refreshing sleep. One may train oneself to sleep in spite of more or less noise. Yet the more quiet and peaceful the surroundings, the easier it becomes to arrive at a condition of complete mental and nervous relaxation. Sounds tend to excite the nervous reactions, which are disturbing.

In the same way, light interferes with restful sleep, for even though the eyes may be closed the lids are not entirely light-proof and a certain amount of light penetrates. This light is more or less stimulating and prevents absolute relaxation of the optic nerves. Complete darkness is much more conducive to sound sleep and, for this reason, one should avoid having any light best that one should retire fairly early in the evening and rise early in the morning. Sleep in the late morning, during several hours of daylight, is not conducive to complete rest. "Early to bed and early to rise," may not make a man wealthy and wise, according to the old saying, but it unquestionably does have some relation to making him healthy.

Fresh air is even more important than darkness or quiet as a factor in inducing restful sleep. The need for oxygen during the building-up processes of sleep is self-evident, but the influence of fresh air *as a means of enabling one to sleep more soundly* is not always appreciated. If you want to know what truly refreshing sleep, beginning as soon as the head touches the pillow, really is, try sleeping out of doors. The next thing to that is sleeping in a room with several windows wide open, so as to approximate the condition of outdoor life as nearly as possible.

In winter bodily warmth is a necessary factor in sleep. The feet, particularly, should be thoroughly warm. On the other hand, an overheated condition is always conducive to restlessness. Do not cover too heavily. The nerve pressure incidental to heavy coverings is disturbing. In other words, while warmth is necessary, one should have no more covering than is absolutely required to maintain warmth. Cotton blankets and quilts are extremely heavy, but have little warmth. Wool is light and, whether in the form of blankets or wool-filled quilts, is ideal for cold-weather use. Down comforters likewise provide warmth without weight. During the hot summer nights it is best to sleep absolutely without covering and sometimes even without any night apparel.

A reasonably hard bed with a good, firm mattress is preferable to undue softness of bedding. If one lies on one's back, it would certainly be better not to use a pillow. A pillow is likewise unnecessary if one sleeps on the chest, so to speak, or partially on one side. This is probably the best position for sound and refreshing sleep. If one sleeps on the side, then a pillow is desirable for comfort.

The best remedy for sleeplessness is probably a hot foot bath, as it draws the blood away from the brain. This treatment may be supplemented by cold cloths applied to the forehead in case of mental stimulation, emotional excitement or congestion of the brain due to any cause. A drink of hot water or hot milk will draw the blood from the brain to the stomach.

A condition of normal muscular fatigue is always favorable to slumber, and if you have taken the exercises described in another chapter and spent sufficient time out of doors either in walking or in any other exercise, you can almost depend upon a condition of healthy fatigue that will enable you to sleep well.

The air bath is another invaluable means of soothing the nervous system and bringing about a condition favorable to sleep. Simply remove all clothing for a half hour before going to bed, providing the room is not too cold.

In many cases a walk in the open air just before bedtime is to be recommended. Although walking for the purpose of exercise should be brisk and vigorous in order to be beneficial, the walk before bedtime for the sake of inducing sleep will be more effective if taken at a leisurely gait, especially if deep breathing is practiced during a good part of the walk.

CHAPTER XXIV:
Fresh Air, Bathing and
Other Health Factors ▲

It goes without saying that an outdoor nation will be infinitely more rugged than a race of people that lives chiefly indoors. We may not be altogether an indoor race, but we are far too much so. Great numbers of people can measure the average amount of time spent daily in the open air in minutes, whereas it should be measured in hours.

Outdoor life is one of the most potent of all factors in maintaining and restoring health. Pure outdoor air has a tonic effect upon the digestion, upon the quality of the blood, upon the nerves, upon the brain and upon the entire organism. Fresh air in large quantities is one of the first essentials to health.

Every one should make it a point, therefore, to spend a certain part of each day in the open air, irrespective of the weather. It is not sufficient to spend fifteen minutes or a half hour out of doors. You should make it two or three hours at the very least, and more if possible. Many people will object that they can not find time for such a purpose, but often it will be found that they devote more than the two or three hours in question to indoor recreation of one kind or another. It is a very simple plan to choose outdoor recreations in place of those taken indoors. Even motoring is commendable because it takes one into the open air.

The practice of bathing is one of the marks of civilization, although primitive peoples instinctively take to the water when they have the opportunity through pure enjoyment of the bath. Bathing has two functions. It serves as a means of cleanliness and as a tonic.

Cold baths may be said to be chiefly tonic in their influence. They are stimulating. They have a pronounced effect upon circulation, and may be useful in strengthening the heart. They have, however, very little cleansing value, unless used in combination with plenty of soap.

A cold bath offers an ideal means of waking one up and toning up the nervous system, as well as arousing or stimulating an active circulation. In this respect it may supplement any exercise that one may take each morning. The cold bath should always follow the exercises which warm one up to such a degree that the sensation of the cold water upon the skin is a pleasure.

The benefit of a cold bath may be measured in a general way by the pleasure one finds in it. If the bath is something in the nature of an ordeal, if one dreads it and feels thoroughly chilled both during and after the experience, then it can not be of any value. To those who are of too frail a constitution to be able to react or recuperate from a cold bath, it can not be recommended. It is absolutely necessary that one should react with the feeling of warmth and comfort immediately after.

Unless you arc fairly rugged, therefore, do not attempt a cold bath except when you feel thoroughly warm, and can take it in a warm room. See that your hands and feet arc not cold. Preliminary exercise is usually desirable for the sake of insuring thorough warmth. Following a hot bath also one is naturally disposed to enjoy cold water and a quick cold sponging or shower is usually desirable at such a time to close the pores.

A cold tub or cold shower will offer a rather strenuous form of cold bathing. If you are not vigorous enough for such measures, then try a sponge bath, if necessary, sponging only one part of the body at a time. A fairly good plan, if your recuperative powers are weak, is to take a preliminary hot foot bath, or to stand with the feet in hot water while taking a cold sponge. Do not try to use water that is too cold in the beginning. Use water of a moderate temperature at first and gradually accustom yourself to a colder bath. You will find it a delightful tonic when you have once hardened your body in such a way that you can thoroughly enjoy it.

A warm bath in soap and water is valuable not only for cleanliness, but for its quieting and soothing effect upon the nerves. A hot bath, in which classification may be placed any bath from 102 degrees up to 110 degrees, is very effective for breaking up a cold and for eliminating poisons from the system, in kidney trouble and various other diseases. A cabinet steam bath, or dry hot-air bath, will, to a large extent, serve the same purpose as a regular Turkish bath, but if a cabinet is unavailable an improvised Turkish bath may be arranged by means of a hot foot bath taken in a warm room while wrapped in blankets. Drinking hot water or hot lemonade will help. The hot water bath will, however, answer just as well in many cases and is far more convenient. It is best to use a bath thermometer so that you can determine the temperature beforehand.

Air baths and sun baths are tonics of no small value, especially so far as the nervous system is concerned. Modern methods of clothing tend too much to smother the skin. Let your skin breathe. An air bath of half an hour or longer before going to bed, or at any other time of the day that may be convenient, will have a tonic effect upon the entire nervous system, besides stimulating the activity of the pores. The same is even more true of a sun bath. A little sunshine each day is almost a necessity. It may be said, however, that those of exceedingly fair skin should be careful not to expose themselves too much to the noonday sun in midsummer. The rays of the sun may be as harmful to blondes as they are beneficial to others.

A dry friction rub constitutes another very stimulating and refreshing form of dry bathing. This may be applied either with soft flesh brushes, a rough Turkish towel, or by vigorous rubbing of the entire body with the bare hands. Five minutes of this will have a splendid tonic effect, improving the circulation and also the smoothness and texture of the skin.

The condition of the skin and the care of the skin are important because this wonderful covering of the body is not merely an external coating, but an organ with very important functions. The skin constitutes one of the channels of elimination. Its health and activity are necessary to keep the blood pure. It is related to the nervous system in a most important way; our sense of touch is dependent upon its millions of infinitesimal nerve endings. Through the power of contraction or relaxation of this wonderful surface of the body, the circulation is controlled and the body enabled to adapt itself to the varying changes of the temperature. It will be seen, therefore, how and why the care of the skin is important.

For all these reasons the clothing that we wear has a decided effect upon the general health. The more porous it is, admitting the free circulation of air upon the surface of the body, the more satisfactory and healthful it will be found. Avoid tightly woven or airtight garments. They do not permit of the "ventilation" of the skin. The loosely woven fabrics are also much warmer.

A very good general rule is never to wear any more clothing than is absolutely necessary. This does not mean that in severe winter weather one should go about in a chilled condition. It is better, however, to depend upon a good circulation for warmth than upon excessive clothing, or bed covering. In summer, the more nearly your clothing enables you to enjoy a continuous air bath the better.

Open-mesh linen or cotton underwear is especially recommended for summer. For those who work indoors heavy underwear is probably undesirable at any time of year, for the reason that homes and offices are usually heated to a summer temperature. Comfort outdoors should be secured by using sweaters, gaiters and overcoats.

Another factor in clothing of some importance and interest is the question of color. Black and dark-colored fabrics shut out the light, whereas white, tan, light gray and other light-colored goods permit the light to penetrate, thus giving one a light bath, so to speak, when in the sunshine. Light-colored clothes are superior for summer wear for the additional reason that they are cool. White and light-colored materials reflect the heat and transmit the light. Dark-colored clothes absorb the heat, but do not transmit the light. Black clothing in the sunshine is very hot indeed. It may be advantageous in winter for this reason. Some students of this and allied health problems have adopted the practice of wearing tan-colored or other light clothing the year round, holding that even during the evening the body receives some benefit from the electric light-rays.

CHAPTER XXV:
Eye Hygiene ▲

Much that has been written about the care of the eyes is erroneous and misleading. We have been exhorted not to read in bed, and told with much detail just how the various positions in which the body and the book must be held disarranged our internal machinery. We have been warned against reading on the train, the only place, in many cases, where people have time to read. Even that delightful practice, reading at meals, has been condemned in unmeasured terms. We have been instructed as to the distance which should intervene between reading matter and the eyes, and even the angle at which the book we are reading, or the paper on which we are writing, should be adjusted. The effect of light has been discussed endlessly, and we have been warned against the evil effects both of too much and too little.

We have been told that reading was a dangerous practice at best, and that, if we must read, we should, as we valued our eyesight, avoid fine print, although the types of the newspapers are among those classed as too small to be safe in large quantities and we can't live without reading newspapers.

Most of us pay no attention to any of these instructions, reading when, where and how we please and can, and therefore, it is gratifying to learn that none of them have any material bearing upon the preservation of our sight. The essential thing is to learn how to use the eyes properly. Then all such details as the foregoing can safely be left to the inclination and convenience of the individual.

In the case of light there is much evidence to show that the views commonly held have no basis in fact.

Rabbit's eyes have been exposed to the most intense light known, avoiding heat, but subsequent examination of the eyes with the microscope revealed no change either in the retina, the optic nerve, or the brain. A teacher of fifteen years' experience complained that because her classroom was in the basement and the light poor, the sight of her pupils was worse at the end of every school year than it was at the beginning. The classrooms where the light was good, however, had the same experience; and when the Snellen test card was introduced into both the well-lighted and the poorly-lighted classrooms, and the children used it every day, the sight of all improved, regardless of lighting conditions. In Germany it was demonstrated by the statistics of Cohn and others that improvements in the lighting of the schools made in the hope of staying the progress of myopia did not have that effect.

These and other observations show that poor lighting has very little, if anything, to do with the production of eye defects.

The fact is that anyone who can read comfortably in a poor light is to be congratulated, and need not be afraid to continue the practice. If he were straining his eyes, he could not do it, whereas in a good light one can read in spite of the strain.

People who have perfect sight think very little about the light, but it is undoubtedly more comfortable to have it so arranged that no shadow is thrown upon the work, either from the head, hand, or any other object, and so that it shines upon the page which one is reading, or upon the desk at which one is writing, not into the eyes.

Protection of the eyes from strong light is not necessary. In fact, the light is beneficial, as we have already demonstrated. The glare from snow or water may be trying, and smoked or amber glasses will conduce to comfort, but, ordinarily, no harm will be done if they are not worn.

Since the moving pictures came in we have heard much about the strain imposed upon the eyes by this new appurtenance of civilization, and predictions of dire results to our already very bad eyesight, in consequence of our constant attendance upon these exhibitions, have been made. Theoretically, this view of the matter seems a reasonable one. The ordinary rate at which the film runs through the projecting machine is about a foot a second—sixteen pictures a second. That is to say, sixteen distinct pictures are thrown upon the screen in each second of time, and the shutter comes down and is raised that number of times each second also. Between each projected picture there must be a black period, for if this were not the case, the pictures would all run into one another, in a hopeless blur.

It might have been expected that these rapid alternations of light and darkness would be very trying to the eyes, and they often do produce much temporary discomfort, particularly in persons suffering from errors of refraction. Some years ago when the mechanical process involved was less perfect than it has since become, the strain was probably much greater than it is now. Today there is no reason for supposing that the movies are injurious to the eyes. On the contrary they have been found to be a great benefit. Instead of avoiding them, persons who do not suffer from them should go to them frequently, and those who do should accustom their eyes to them gradually, at the same time practicing the methods recommended in this book for the improvement of the vision. Often all that is necessary to relieve the strain is to close the eyes frequently, or look away from the screen, while viewing the pictures.

As for the dangers of fine print, those who understand the principles of central fixation will understand that it is easier, normally, to see small things than larger ones, and that the fear of fine print is, therefore, as baseless as the fear of light.

The fact is that the eye is a much less fragile instrument than we have generally supposed it to be. If properly used, it is fully able to withstand all the strains of modern life.

CHAPTER XXVI:
Test Your Own Eyes ▲

It does not require any special training, or even any expensive apparatus, to test the vision. With the aid of a Snellen test card any one can test his own sight, and with the assistance of a second person a retinoscope can be used.

A test card, which is sometimes difficult to buy, accompanies this course. You can also make one for yourself by painting black letters of an appropriate size on a white background. Directions for using the card for the purpose of testing the vision are given in Chapter XI, "Saving the Sight of the Children." Each eye should, of course, be tested separately.

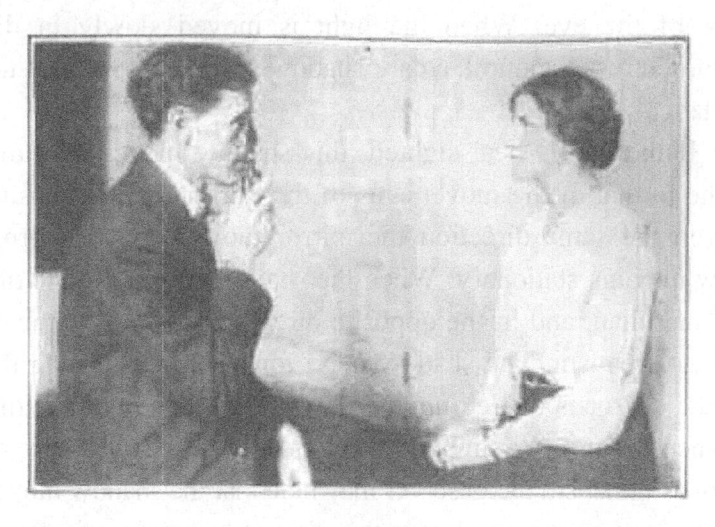

26-1. Testing the eye with the retinoscope. ▲

A retinoscope can be even more easily made than a test card, all the material required for the purpose being a small piece of looking-glass about one inch wide and three inches long. A small mirror that will answer the purpose can be bought at the five-and-ten-cent stores, and a glass-cutter, which is as easy to use as a pair of scissors, can also be bought at these stores. For a few cents, too, a glazier, or painter, will cut a piece of mirror glass of the right size. About three-quarters of an inch from the top of this mirror, and midway between the sides, scrape off the silver backing on an area a little larger than the lead of a lead-pencil. If it is a little larger, or a little smaller than this, it will not matter. By means of the mirror the observer reflects light from a lamp, or other source of light, into the eye which is being examined, and the opening serves as a sight-hole through which he looks into the pupil. The room must be darkened, and the light placed a little behind and over the head of the subject.

When the observer, who stands or is seated a few feet from the subject, looks through the sight-hole, he observes that the pupil, instead of being black, is more or less red. This is the color of the retina, which is not ordinarily seen, because the eye of the observer is not placed in position to receive the rays of light coming from the interior of the eye. When the light is moved slowly in different directions across the pupil, a dark shadow will be observed at the edge of the latter.

If the eye is near-sighted, this shadow moves in a direction opposite to that of the movements of the mirror. If it is far-sighted it moves in the same direction the mirror moves. If it is normal, the shadow remains stationary. When the shadow moves in one direction in one meridian, and in the opposite direction in another, the eye has mixed astigmatism. The shadow may, for instance, go with the light when the mirror is moved up and down, and in an opposite direction to it when the mirror is moved from side to side. In the case of other kinds of astigmatism the observer may note that the shadow moves more decidedly in one meridian than in the other. When errors of refraction are corrected by glasses there will be no movement of the shadow.

The retinoscope can be used as an ophthalmoscope simply by lessening the distance between the observer and the subject. The principle is just the same as that involved in looking through a keyhole into a room. The closer you come to the keyhole the more you will see. At a distance of about half an inch, by looking a little toward the nasal side of the eye, one will begin to see the optic nerve, an area whiter than the rest of the interior of the eyeball and apparently about one-quarter of an inch in diameter. Radiating from the center one sees fine streaks of branching blood vessels, the darker being the veins, the lighter the arteries.

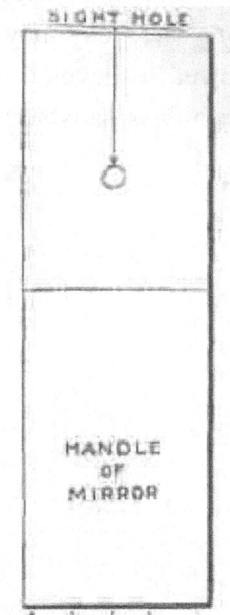

26-2. A simple homemade retinoscope, made by scratching a small hole in the silver back of a small mirror, to be used for self-testing in conjunction with another larger mirror. ▲

It requires no experience to make these observations, and children of ten have used the instrument successfully. The larger the pupil the easier it is, just as in the case of the keyhole. The larger the opening the more one sees in both cases. The normal eye is more easily examined than a defective one, and young adults than older or younger persons. The light should be thrown on the blind spot, the entrance of the optic nerve, as the pupil contracts when it is thrown on the center of sight. The red light should be seen constantly in the pupil. When it is lost the observer should withdraw a little and get it again, afterward bringing the instrument up close to the eye.

There are also various other ways in which the vision can be tested. If the subject, when looking at the letters on the Snellen test card, can remember anything blacker, the vision is imperfect, no matter what the light, or the distance. Another way is to squint the eyes, or to look through a small opening, such as a hole in a card, or an opening between the fingers. If this enables you to see better, your vision is imperfect.

Everyone should have the means of making these simple tests, for eye troubles when not accompanied by discomfort, are insidious, and may make considerable progress before they are discovered. This is particularly apt to be the case if one eye is principally affected. So long as one has one fairly good eye to see with one may not observe that the other is falling behind, and when an eye once begins to do this it can hardly fail to lose function rapidly, simply because it does not get enough work to do. If errors of refraction are discovered at the beginning, they can be quickly corrected by the methods presented in this book; but if they are allowed to continue for years, they may be very difficult to cure. And if the eye is not allowed to develop any permanent errors of refraction and the general health is satisfactory, one need have no fear of organic diseases.

CHAPTER XXVII:
A Final Word
to Those Who Wear Glasses ▲

Persons coming to this country from Europe are always struck by the number of people using artificial aids to vision, for the United States seems to have pre-empted the position formerly held by Germany as the land of the eyeglass. Thousands of people in this country wear glasses whose vision for reading and distance is normal without them. What more they could expect of their eyes and why they wear glasses it is difficult to understand. They will tell you that glasses remove strain, enable them to read longer, or to do work that their eyes could not be expected to do without them. The fact is, as has been explained, that glasses can never remove strain, but must, on the contrary, be a cause of strain. It is also a fact that glasses, though fitted by the best of oculists, can never give as good vision as the normal eye enjoys without them.

Or they will tell you that they put on glasses in the first place because they were subject to frequent headaches, and as the pain was above the eyes, they were convinced that they were due to eye strain. This may have been true, because a very slight error of refraction will sometimes cause a great deal of discomfort. But the trouble may have been a temporary one that would have passed away if the patient had not resorted to glasses, and headaches may be due to many things besides eye strain: improper diet, indigestion, constipation, lack of fresh air, insufficient exercise and too little sleep being the usual causes. Glasses have probably caused a great many more headaches than they have cured, and an oculist's prescription for those conditions is extremely illogical. A correction of their harmful, energy-dissipating habits of living would soon convince the majority of such persons that there was little or nothing wrong with their eyes. All that stands between them and eye freedom, probably, is a few days of discomfort, the natural consequence of the readjustment to ocular self-dependence.

Whether the vision is normal or not, everyone who wears glasses should discard them as quickly as possible, and those who understand the facts will surely not delay a day longer than is necessary in doing so. It can be done in all but a very few cases, and has been done by thousands. If one makes his living by the use of his eyes, and cannot see to do his work without glasses he cannot, obviously, discard the latter at once, but some people are able to make progress in spite of this handicap, reducing the strength of the lenses as their refraction improves, if necessary, while others may be able to make the necessary start during a vacation. The transition from glasses to no-glasses may be unpleasant, but usually the discomfort is not serious, and if glasses can be completely discarded, does not last long. The wearing of glasses for work and other necessary purposes is a complication that had better be eliminated if it is in any way possible, because the refraction may change very quickly, and we all know how uncomfortable it is to put on glasses not adapted to our eyes for even a moment. Myopic persons have a great advantage in the fact that they can see at the near-point without their glasses, and near vision is the kind most needed under modern conditions. Hypermetropic persons can often see well enough at the near-point to read without glasses, but are more likely to have headaches when they first try to get on without them than are the myopic.

Most people heartily dislike glasses, because of their effect on personal appearance, their inconvenience, and the imperfect vision secured through their use. Persons who have worn them for any length of time know by the evidence of their own senses that their eyes have grown steadily weaker under their influence. That the conditions for which they are worn are curable cannot be disputed by any one who will impartially examine the facts. Yet, most people cannot be persuaded to give the new way a trial. Ignoring even the facts of their own experience, they cling to their glasses for fear they may lose their eyesight if they go without them. The process of cure, moreover, is often tedious, though in the majority of cases it takes only a moderate amount of time, and many people would rather put up with the inconvenience of glasses than make the necessary effort to get rid of them.

For all these reasons the gospel of no-glasses spreads slowly, and opticians who have accepted it say they have no fear of its injuring business.

There remains, however, a considerable minority who insist on doing their own thinking, no matter how much their conclusions may be opposed to the teaching of tradition and authority, and who are willing to take as much trouble as may be necessary to preserve that most precious of all possessions, their sight. To them this book is addressed, and on them we must depend to lead the way where a new generation will follow.

[THE END]

ABOUT THE ORIGINAL AUTHOR

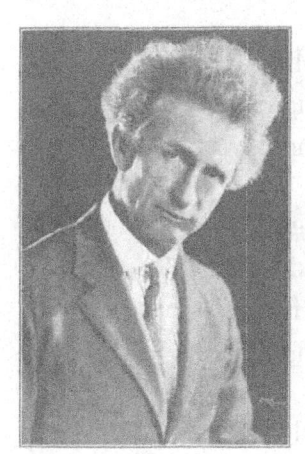

Bernarr Macfadden *(born Bernard Adolphus McFadden, August 16, 1868 – October 12, 1955)* was an American proponent of physical culture, a combination of bodybuilding with nutritional and health theories. He also founded the long-running magazine publishing company Macfadden Publications. He was the predecessor of Charles Atlas and Jack LaLanne, and has been credited with beginning the culture of health and fitness in the United States.

Macfadden popularized the practice of fasting that previously had been associated with illnesses such as anorexia nervosa. He felt strongly that fasting was one of the surest ways to physical health. Many of his subjects would fast for a week in order to rejuvenate their body. He claimed that "a person could exercise unqualified control over virtually all types of disease while revealing a degree of strength and stamina such as would put others to shame" through fasting. He saw fasting as an instrument with which to prove a man's superiority over other men.

APPENDIX & RESOURCES

I Can See Clearly Now 132
Snellen Eye Chart 133
Snellen Fraction Explained 134
Eye Can See Clearly Now Infographic 136
Who is the Ageless Adept? 137
Books in the Ageless Adept Series 138
Free Resources 139
Channels & Blogs 140
Vitality Tests & Quizzes 140
T-Shirts, Mugs & More 140

I CAN SEE CLEARLY NOW

I can see clearly now, the rain has gone
I can see all obstacles in my way
Gone are the dark clouds that had me blind
It's gonna be a bright, bright sun-shining day
It's gonna be a bright, bright sun-shining day

I think I can make it now, the pain has gone
All of the bad feelings have disappeared
Here is that rainbow I've been praying for
It's gonna be a bright, bright sun-shining day

Look all around, there's nothing but blue sky
Look straight ahead, nothing but blue sky

I can see clearly now, the rain has gone
I can see all obstacles in my way
Gone're the dark clouds that had me blind
It's gonna be a bright, bright sun-shining day
It's gonna be a bright, bright sun-shining day
Gonna be a bright, bright sun-shining day
Gonna be a bright, bright, bright sun-shining day
Lyrics by Johnny Nash

SNELLEN EYE CHART▲

E	1	20/200
F P	2	20/100
T O Z	3	20/70
L P E D	4	20/50
P E C F D	5	20/40
E D F C Z P	6	20/30
F E L O P Z D	7	20/25
D E F P O T E C	8	20/20
L E F O D P C T	9	
F D P L T C E O	10	
P E Z O L C F T D	11	

A typical Snellen chart developed by Dutch ophthalmologist Herman Snellen in 1862, to estimate visual acuity. When printed out at the correct size, the E on line one will be 88.7 mm (3.5 inches) and the letters on the 20/20 line should be 8.87 millimeters tall. When viewed at a distance of 20 ft (= 609.6 centimeters, or 6.09600 meters), you can estimate your eyesight based on the smallest line you are able to read.

Download free at www.agelessadept.com/resources

SNELLEN FRACTION EXPLAINED▲

An ophthalmologist referring to your visual acuity may say, *"You have 20/20 [or 20/10] vision,"* using what's called a Snellen Fraction, named after Herman Snellen. Let's explore exactly what that means.

The Snellen fraction is defined as: *A representation of visual acuity in the form of a fraction (e.g. 20/20 (6/6), 20,80 (6/24), etc.) in which the numerator is the testing distance, usually expressed in feet (or meters), and the denominator is the distance at which the smallest Snellen letter readable by the eye "has an angular size of 5 minutes."* [or, alternatively: *[the letter] "subtends a visual angle of 5 minutes of arc (written 5') at the eye.*]

That can all be a bit confusing. So, here's what it all means:

1. First, the reason the number "20" is used in these measurements is because, in the U.S., the standard length of an eye exam room (the distance from patient to acuity chart) is about 20 feet. *(In countries where meters are used instead of feet, a typical eye exam room is about 6 meters long. Six meters is 19.685 feet, which is close enough to 20 feet for use. Therefore, instead 20/20 for normal vision, a notation of 6/6 can be used.)*

2. In geometry, angle size is measured in degrees and minutes (eg. 35° 12' is read as "thirty five degrees, 12 minutes") (Note: 1 degree = 60 minutes). The 5 minute angle size (0° 5') is simply a size that Snellen found to be most conducive to easy reading at 20 feet.

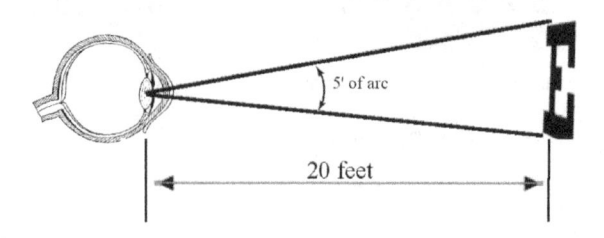

3. If the fraction is 1 or *more* (that is, if the *denominator* (bottom number) is equal to or *less than* than 20; *20/20, 20/15, 20/10*), then your vision is **normal to better than normal!** *The smaller the denominator, the better your vision.*

If the fraction is 1 or *less* (that is, if the *denominator* (bottom number) is *more* than 20; *20/30, 20/40, 20/50*), then your vision is **in need of rejuvenation.** *The larger the denominator, the worse your vision.*

Here are some graphics to help you visualize and remember what the Snellen Fraction means:

$$\frac{20}{10} =$$

Translation: "At twenty feet, the smallest letters I can read are what they need to move closer to 10 feet to see! My vision is 20/10 or 2X normal! Yippee!"

$$\frac{20}{50} =$$

Translation: "At 20 ft, the smallest letters I can read are letters they can see from 50 feet. My vision is 20/50 or 2/5 of normal. Bummer."

Editor's Source: Developed with help from the best explanation I've found on the web: *Anatomy, Physiology & Pathology of the Human Eye* www.tedmontgomery.com/the_eye/acuity.html

The Eye Can See Clearly Infographic

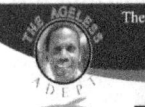

The Ageless Adept, publisher of *Fast & Grow Young* presents

How to Reclaim Your Vision and Keep Your Eyesight Forever!

The modern re-issue of *Strengthening the Eyes* — A System of Scientific Eye Training By Bernarr Macfadden

Download more free resources at www.agelessadept.com/resources

"...almost every irregularity of the eye can either be cured or materially benefited without the help of glasses."--**Macfadden**

For step-by-step instructions, practice aids, diagrams and much more....
Order the book!
Eye Can See Clearly Now:

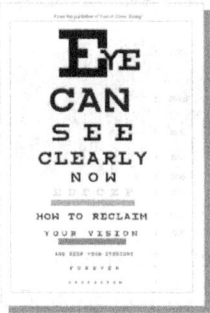

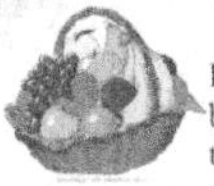

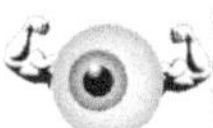

How to reclaim your vision and keep your eyesight forever
by Bernarr Macfadden

1. LEARN TO USE YOUR EYES CORRECTLY
Practice "Central Fixation"
When viewing an object or scene, do not attempt to see everything all at once. Instead, focus only on one point. You'll see the image sharper and clearer with less strain. This is called "central fixation." The goal of training your eyes in this way is to develop the habit of *seeing without strain*--the key to maintaining your eyesight!

2. WORK YOUR EYE MUSCLES
Do the 5 minute "Eyebo" Workout
Muscles control the eyes. Astigmatism, Near-far sightedness, and other conditions are "...due to the abnormal action of the muscles and.. their cure is therefore a mere matter of muscular control." These special exercises will have a strengthening and toning-up effect. It's like Tae-bo for the eyes! Call it Eyebo!

3. PRACTICE EYE FOCUSING
Near to far to near to far...
Muscular action accompanies all changes of the focus of the eye, and the power of making these changes must obviously be improved by the daily practice of exercise as well as exercises for the pupil's reaction to dark and light.

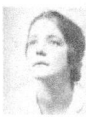

4. SLEEP THE NIGHT AWAY
Get enough health-building, strength-restoring sleep for proper rejuvenation!

5. MASSAGE YOUR EYES
"Hands on" invigoration
Eyes can be strengthened and invigorated by manipulation which quickens the circulation of the blood and stimulates the nerves.

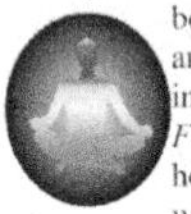

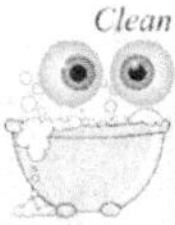

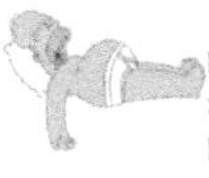

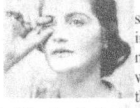

6. BATHE YOUR EYES
Clean eyes=clean sight!
Use an eye cup or simple basin for bathing the eyes in a weak solution of salt water.

7. EXERCISE THE BODY
"I like to move it!"
These 25 movements will "...increase the oxygen intake until your entire body from top to toe is charged with it. This will make you more alive. It will make you brighter and more energetic, and the improved circulation will tend to tone up every cell and every structure of the body."

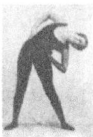

8. EAT REAL FOOD
Food nourishes the blood. Blood nourishes the eyes. Eat only unmodified, organic, non-GMO, chemical-free fruits and vegetables in as close to their natural state as possible....only when hungry!

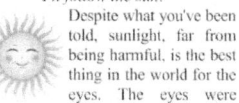

9. SEEK SUNLIGHT
"I'll follow the sun!"
Despite what you've been told, sunlight, far from being harmful, is the best thing in the world for the eyes. The eyes were made to react to light, and in its absence they deteriorate and become weak.

10. FAST & GROW YOUNG!
The body is coded to heal
Fasting for extended periods lets the body purge, detox, heal and rejuvenate the body including the eyes. Read *Fast & Grow Young* for how to do an extended water fast correctly!

© *Eye Can See Clearly Now*, published by Walt F.J. Goodridge. Print/Share freely!

All products and freebies on the following pages available at

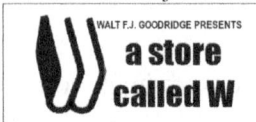

WALT F.J. GOODRIDGE PRESENTS
a store called W

A STORE CALLED W!
www.waltgoodridge.com/store
Eye'll see you there!

Who is the Ageless Adept? ▲

"Perfect health, long life and eternal youth are not the random, genetic blessings of a chaotic or capricious universe, but natural birthrights that can be accessed through the mindful acceptance of simple truths, activated by the disciplined practice of proven protocols, and sustained by advancement along a known path. This is that path."

My name is Walt F.J. Goodridge, author and publisher of the *Ageless Adept*™ series of books, and I'm here to prove a point!

Years ago, before I became vegan, a friend—over lunch--asked a question over lunch I couldn't answer: *"Do you know what's in the food you're eating?"* I did not, and as a trained engineer, it bothered me that I had failed such a simple test, and so--with health, longevity and vitality as my goals--I dedicated my life to a search for answers and ultimately to *"share what I know, so that others may grow."*

My childhood in the Caribbean steeped in me an understanding of and reverence for our natural world of sunshine, water, earth, air and time. As an adult, I discovered that what passes as *normal* health and healing in the western paradigm is shockingly *unnatural*! It never made sense to me that natural beings should need to turn to men in lab coats with little pills in search of wellness. It makes more sense that Nature would have the answers built in; that our bodies would have an innate healing code; that our "operations manual" would be simple and foolproof.

Through my own experiments, the testimonials of others of like mind, and the corroboration of researchers from this and previous eras, I've realized that the symptoms we as a society accept as a "normal" part of aging are simply the body's reactions to unnatural habits of ingesting pharmaceuticals, fake food with non-food ingredients, pesticides, hormones, steroids and antibiotics, as well as other environmental factors. Some of the causes (i.e., habits) may be hard to break, but are ultimately under our control and controllable. And, if the *causes* are controllable, then the *effects* are not inevitable and may even be reversible! That's what I'm here to prove!

I've distilled the results of my experiments into my Ageless Adept™ philosophy and protocols--information I hope will (1) empower you to become your own authority in matters of health, and (2) make better survival decisions choosing from among the products and practices you'll encounter on your own path of perfect health, long life and the fountain of youth!

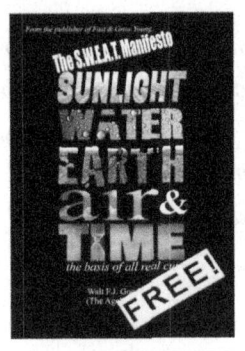

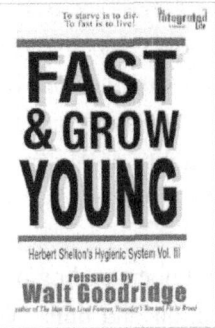

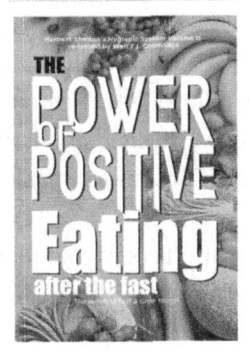

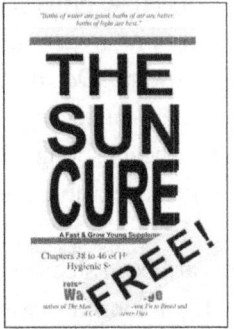

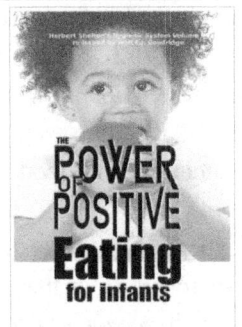

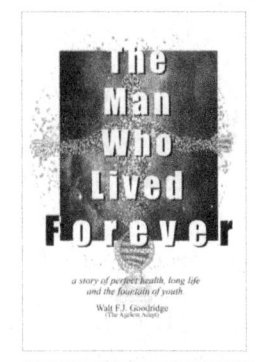

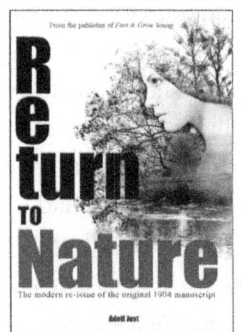

Books in the Ageless Adept Series ▲

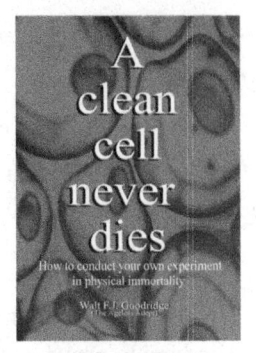

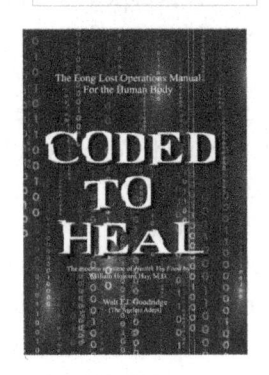

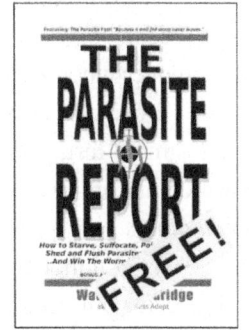

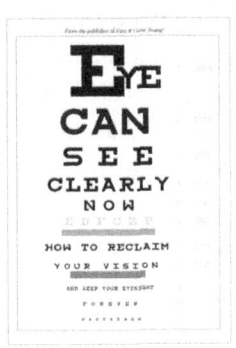

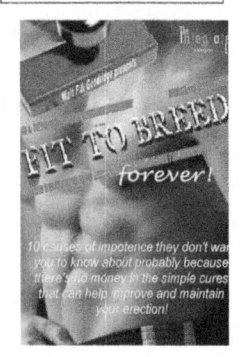

Free resources are available at www.waltgoodridge.com/store

More Ageless Adept Resources ▲

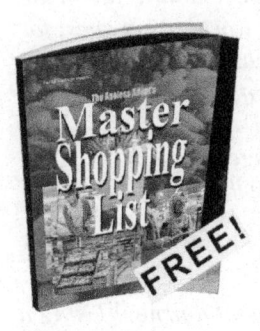

The Ageless Adept's Master Shopping List, Substitution Checklist & Immunity Top 10

What do I, the Ageless Adept, buy when going grocery shopping? What's in my spice rack? What healthy condiments do I keep on hand? What kind of juicer did I get? Want to see my colloidal silver generator? Yes, I have a coffee grinder (for enemas only, of course!)

Here are the supplements, tools and toys I have on hand at all times--even when I travel--that fit in with the Clean Cell lifestyle and keep me on the path of perfect health, long life and the fountain of youth!

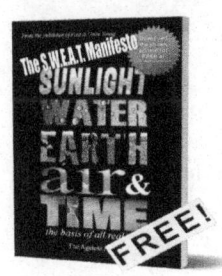

The S.W.E.A.T. Manifesto

The basis of REAL cure—treatment that actually ELIMINATES illness—must & always will require incorporating the power of **S**unlight, **W**ater, **E**arth, **A**ir or **T**ime. (S.W.E.A.T.) This is *The S.W.E.A.T. Manifesto.*

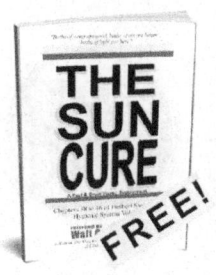

The Sun Cure

The Sun Cure is the re-issue of chapters 38 to 46 of Shelton's Hygienic System Vol II. These chapters from the original text were not included in *Fast & Grow Young*. Shelton explores and explains the numerous physiological, psychological and emotional benefits of direct exposure to sunlight.

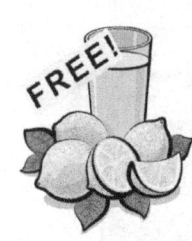

REVITALADE™
A mineral REstorative, VITALity-boosting lemonADE! "The all-natural, great-tasting, made-for-fasting, perfect-for-sauna, microbiome-friendly, energy-enhancing, system-rebooting, mineral-rich, replenisher I developed and have used over the years to live a natural life in an unnatural world!"--The Ageless Adept

Free resources are available at www.waltgoodridge.com/store

Ageless Adept Channels & Blogs ▲

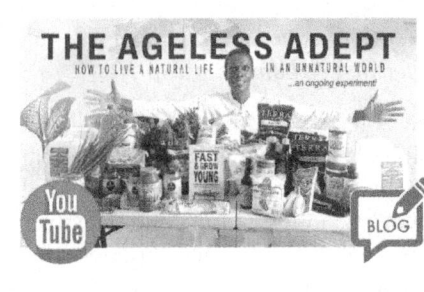

"How I live a natural life in an unnatural world in my quest for perfect health, long life and the fountain of youth!"

Youtube: *@agelessadept*
Blog: *www.agelessadept.com/blog*

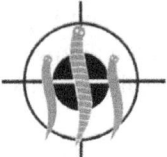

The Parasite Blog: *A recent personal journey: Using a "parasite fast" as part of a comprehensive protocol to eliminate rope worms!*
www.parasiteblog.com

Vitality Tests & Quizzes ▲

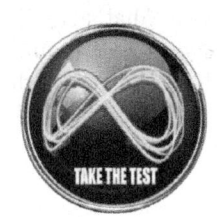

What's your "Longevity Score?"
How will your dietary and lifestyle choices affect your lifespan? Find out!
www.agelessadept.com/longevity-test

Are you "fit to breed?"
Has Nature classified you as worthy to have your DNA passed on to another generation? Take the test!
www.fittobreed.com

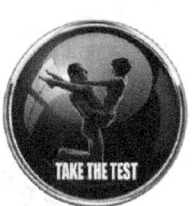

T-Shirts, Mugs & More ▲

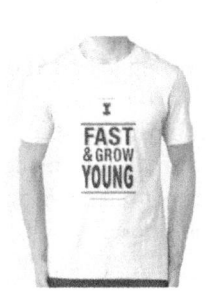

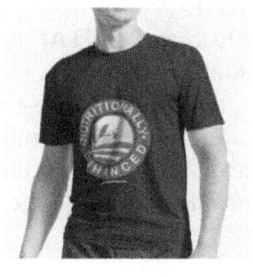

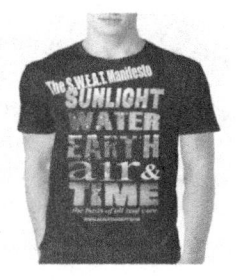

"I Fast & Grow Young" "Nutritionally Enhanced" "Sunlight, Water, Earth, Air & Time" & many more designs available!

Visit https://www.redbubble.com/people/agelessadept

Made in United States
Orlando, FL
30 March 2024